My Neck Hurts!

My Neck Hurts!

Nonsurgical Treatments for Neck and Upper Back Pain

Martin T. Taylor, D.O., Ph.D.

The Johns Hopkins University Press
Baltimore

Note to the Reader: This book embodies a general approach to neck and upper back pain. It was not written about *your specific situation*, and your treatment should not be based solely on what is written here. Your treatment plan must be developed through a dialogue between you and your doctor.

Exercise programs and the use of medications vary from individual to individual. You must first speak with your doctor about your individual needs before beginning any exercise program or using any medications. The exercises described here should be performed first under the supervision of a physical therapist or another professional in exercise therapy.

The author and publisher have exerted every effort to ensure that the selection and dosage of drugs discussed in this text accord with current recommendations and practice at the time of publication. However, in view of ongoing research, changes in governmental regulations, and the constant flow of information relating to drug therapy and drug reactions, the reader is urged to check the package insert of each drug for any change in indications and dosage and for warnings and precautions. This is particularly important when the recommended agent is a new and/or infrequently used drug.

© 2010 Martin T. Taylor, D.O., Ph.D.
All rights reserved. Published 2010
Printed in China on acid-free paper
9 8 7 6 5 4 3 2 1

The Johns Hopkins University Press
2715 North Charles Street
Baltimore, Maryland 21218-4363
www.press.jhu.edu

Library of Congress Cataloging-in-Publication Data
Taylor, Martin T.
   My neck hurts! : nonsurgical treatments for neck and upper back pain / Martin T. Taylor.
      p. cm. — (A Johns Hopkins Press health book)
   Includes index.
   ISBN-13: 978-0-8018-9665-1 (hardcover : alk. paper)
   ISBN-10: 0-8018-9665-7 (hardcover : alk. paper)
   ISBN-13: 978-0-8018-9666-8 (pbk. : alk. paper)
   ISBN-10: 0-8018-9666-5 (pbk. : alk. paper)
   1. Neck pain—Treatment—Popular works. 2. Backache—Treatment—Popular works. 3. Self-care,
Health. I. Title.
   RD771.B217T365 2010
   617.5'3—dc22   2009048740

A catalog record for this book is available from the British Library.

Chapter-opening image for chapter 1 © 2006 Yanik Chauvin; chapter 2 © 2006 Dale Woodall; chapter 5 © 2006 Tyler Olson; chapter 6 © 2006 Douglas McLaughlin; chapter 7 © 2005 Duard van der Westhuizen; chapter 8 © 2005 Ine Beerten; chapter 9 © 2008 Andre Blais. All these images are from BigStockPhoto.com.

Special discounts are available for bulk purchases of this book. For more information, please contact Special Sales at 410-516-6936 or specialsales@press.jhu.edu.

The Johns Hopkins University Press uses environmentally friendly book materials, including recycled text paper that is composed of at least 30 percent post-consumer waste, whenever possible. All of our book papers are acid-free, and our jackets and covers are printed on paper with recycled content.

To my wife, Carisa,
and our children, Ellie Megan, Evan, and Kendall.
All things are possible with your love and inspiration.

To my patients with neck and upper back pain
and to all of those who suffer from this condition.
I hope that this book helps you find
the right treatments and relief.

Contents

Preface

This book was written to empower and educate people who are suffering from chronic neck and upper back pain. Most patients, and even some doctors, are not aware of all the non-surgical options available for treating neck pain. It is my hope that this book will play a role in bringing additional therapeutic options to light for you.

The information in this book will allow you to have an informed discussion with your physician so that together you can make decisions about treatment. Understanding your treatment options can help alleviate the frustration that often accompanies chronic pain. Being as knowledgeable as possible about basic anatomy, the potential causes of pain, and the various treatments available will help you tremendously as you and your doctor discuss your condition and the best way to relieve your symptoms.

As an active participant in these discussions, you can provide valuable information to help your physician develop the best plan for you. Treatment plans are individualized based on many factors, including medical conditions such as arthritis or heart disease—even depression or sleep problems. A carefully developed and individualized treatment plan is far more likely to meet your personal needs and reduce your pain to the greatest extent possible.

Most people experience at least one episode of neck or back pain at some point in their lives. For most of us, that pain will resolve completely within two weeks to three months. Long-term or chronic neck pain is defined as pain that lasts longer than six months. About 14 percent of adults in the United States have chronic neck pain. Whether the pain resolves over the course of six months from the time it starts—or not—it is important to consider an appropriate course of conservative treatment first.

Treatments are considered conservative when they are noninvasive (such as medication) or markedly less invasive than surgery (such as injections). A conservative course of treatment will aim to

- reduce pain and spasm and increase neck range of motion
- assist in managing problems frequently associated with neck pain, such as sleeplessness, depression, anxiety, and moodiness
- improve ability to perform daily activities

Conservative treatment is *not* the first option of choice if you develop symptoms such as loss of bowel or bladder control, progressive weakness in the arms or legs, or profound balance problems. These symptoms may constitute a medical emergency and may require immediate surgery. Surgical emergencies for neck pain are *extremely* rare, however, and most episodes of pain can be successfully treated conservatively.

How long should conservative treatment continue? The answer varies widely. In general, the more pain and dysfunction you experience, the sooner surgical treatments will be considered. The expected post-surgical discomfort or extent of the surgery must also be weighed; for example, microsurgery (small surgery using microscopes) may be considered before fusion, a far more extensive operation. For surgery to be a viable option, a significant anatomical abnormality within the spine must be identified as the major cause of your pain.

If a surgically correctable anatomical reason for a person's neck pain cannot be found, surgery is not an option, and conservative treatment is the only recommended course of action.

This book describes multiple nonsurgical options for the treatment of chronic neck and upper back pain. Your doctor may suggest a combination of treatments for optimal benefit. Different people respond differently to a particular therapy. The side effects of potential treatments also vary. Your input helps determine which treatment is the best fit for you and your lifestyle. Ultimately, the goal of any treatment is to reduce your pain as much as possible. Initial, realistic goals might include a reduction of pain by 50 percent, improvement in quality of life, and improved ability to perform daily activities. Keeping your expectations realistic is important. Remember also that improvement does not always occur in a straight line; pain can improve at some point and yet resurface again later as a result of new physical or emotional stressors. The good news is that many conservative treatments prevent recurrences.

Treatment options are illustrated in patient stories throughout the book. These stories are based on patients I have seen in my own practice or cases that have been shared with me by colleagues. Since I have seen and treated hundreds of patients over the years, it was difficult to choose the examples that space allows in this book. In the end, I chose these stories because they illustrate a number of important points:

- Similar symptoms can result from different pathology and subsequently require different treatment approaches.
- Most patients find that various therapies used in combination are necessary to address chronic pain.
- Persistence is important when pursuing treatment.

I hope you will find this book enlightening and instructive. I have written it to guide you as you investigate and progress through treatment.

Although I recommend that you read the book from beginning to end first, you are also encouraged to continue to dip into it as a resource, as needed. Take it with you when you go to the doctor. You might find that referring to the illustrations while talking with your doctor helps speed understanding—on both sides.

At the end of the book, you will find a list of Web sites where you can learn more about treatments and specialists, as well as the glossary, a quick resource when a technical or medical term seems unfamiliar. Terms defined in the glossary appear in **boldface** type the first time they are discussed.

In my years practicing medicine as a neurologist, it has been my privilege to help hundreds of people suffering from chronic neck and upper back pain find relief and, as a result, an improved quality of life. It is my sincere wish that this book will be one of the elements that helps you achieve the same.

Acknowledgments

Thank you to all those who helped in the editing and creation of this project from beginning to end, including my wife, Carisa, Peggy Gallagher, Mary Kennedy, Ashleigh McKown (assistant editor), Martha Murphy (developmental editor), Melanie Mallon (copyeditor), Julie McCarthy (managing editor), and Courtney Bond (production editor).

Special thanks to Jackie Wehmueller, executive editor at the Johns Hopkins University Press, for believing in this book and making it happen.

Thank you to Angela Darragh, PT, who was instrumental in producing the physical therapy chapter and designing proper exercise protocols.

Thank you to my wife Carisa's ever-present support and understanding as well as her expertise in psychology to help with the sections on counseling the mind-body connection.

Thank you to all of those who acted as models to help illustrate techniques and treatments. Thank you to Emily Pagnotto and Brenda Shoup, who modeled for physical therapy exercises, and to Ronette Young, Brent Magee, Summer McKelvey, Donna Carter, and Matt Amway.

Thank you to my agent Nancy Rosenfeld.

My Neck Hurts!

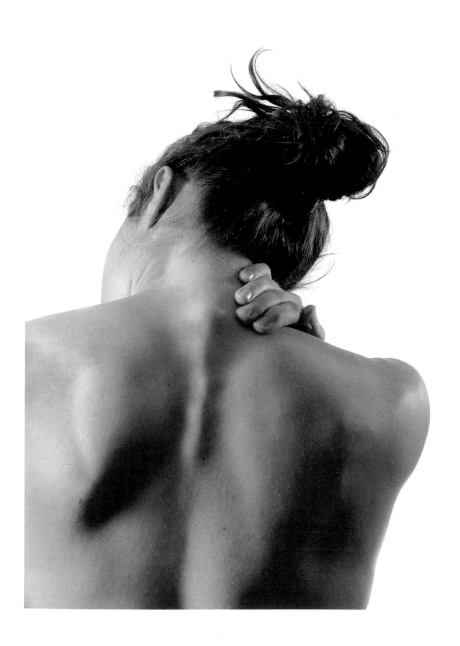

Anatomy of the Neck and Upper Back

What You Need to Know

Understanding the anatomy of the neck and upper back is important before you meet with your doctor to discuss the reasons for the pain you're experiencing and the various options for treatment. You and your doctor can have a more meaningful conversation if you are already familiar with anatomy and with the terms your doctor will use. Better yet, if you prepare a list of observations and questions before your appointment, you will be a more active participant in the decision-making process that lies ahead. By participating in decisions about your treatment, you are likely to experience

3

better results. Bring your list of questions so that you don't have to rely on memory. Also bring a notebook and pen to every appointment. Take notes as your doctor shares information, answers your questions, and makes recommendations.

This chapter provides an overview of spinal anatomy and the major supporting structures and muscles, and can serve as a reference to clarify the following chapters about pathology (disease) and treatments. You can also refer to the glossary at the end of the book for quick definitions.

SPINAL COLUMN

Your spinal column, or "back bone," is made up of a series of bones (**vertebrae**) stacked one on top of another with "shock absorbers" (discs) in between. There are three main sections of the spinal column. These sections are called **cervical, thoracic,** and **lumbar** (see figure 1.1). The **sacrum** and **coccyx** make up the base of the spinal column. They differ from the major vertebrae in that they are fused together and therefore lack **intervertebral discs** (described below). The thoracic, sacral, and coccyx regions gently curve away from the body (**kyphotic**), and the cervical and

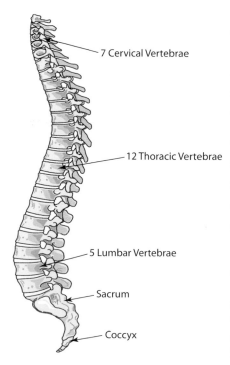

7 Cervical Vertebrae

12 Thoracic Vertebrae

5 Lumbar Vertebrae

Sacrum

Coccyx

FIGURE 1.1   The sections of the spine, showing the seven cervical vertebrae, twelve thoracic vertebrae, five lumbar vertebrae, and the sacrum and coccyx. © 2009 Wolters Kluwer Health | Lippincott Williams and Wilkins.

lumbar regions curve toward the body (**lordotic**). Normal cervical and thoracic curves are approximately 20 to 40 degrees, and a normal lumbar curve is 40 to 60 degrees. These curves help to maintain proper weight distribution in the spine, balance, and flexibility. The vertebrae in each region are numbered, starting with C1 at the top of the cervical spine (C1–C7), T1–T12 in the thoracic region, and L1–L5 in the lumbar region.

SPINAL CORD AND NERVE ROOTS

The **spinal cord** extends from the base of the brain to the area between the bottom of the first lumbar vertebra and the top of the second lumbar vertebra. The spinal cord ends by dividing into individual nerves that travel out to the lower body and legs. This group of nerves at the end of the spinal cord is called the *cauda equine* (the Latin name for a horse's tail). For a short distance, these **nerve roots** travel through the spinal canal before they exit the neural foramen (figure 1.2).

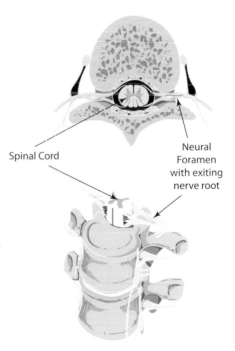

Spinal Cord

Neural Foramen with exiting nerve root

Your spinal cord is protected by the dura mater, a membrane that forms a watertight sack around the spinal cord and nerves. This sack is filled with fluid (**cerebrospinal fluid**), which helps protect the

FIGURE 1.2   Cross-section of the spinal cord. © 2009 Wolters Kluwer Health | Lippincott Williams and Wilkins.

spinal cord from trauma and infection. The nerves in each area of the spinal cord connect to specific parts of the body. In the cervical spine (your neck), for example, the nerves control the upper chest and arms. The nerves also carry signals and sensations back to the brain. Damage to or irritation of the nerves, nerve roots, or spinal cord can lead to pain, tingling, numbness, and weakness.

VERTEBRAE

The vertebrae are the bones that give your spine its structural support. Each vertebra forms a bony ring, which is distinguished by three parts: the **vertebral body,** which is the largest part of the bone (also referred to as the **anterior,** or front); the **laminae,** which are smaller and flank

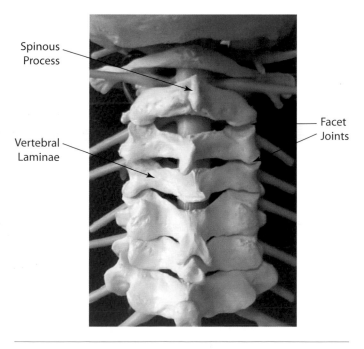

FIGURE 1.3   Posterior view of the vertebrae of the neck (cervical vertebrae).

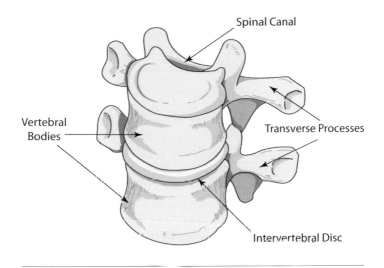

Spinal Canal

Vertebral Bodies

Transverse Processes

Intervertebral Disc

FIGURE 1.4   A section of the spine forming the spinal canal.
© 2009 Wolters Kluwer Health | Lippincott Williams and Wilkins.

the bony **posterior** (back) of your spine; and the **spinous process,** which you can feel with your fingertips, running down the center of your back (see figure 1.3).

The central area formed by this ring is called the **central canal**, or spinal canal, and it contains and protects the spinal cord. Bony protrusions, called **transverse processes**, extend on both sides of the ring (figure 1.4).

The vertebrae in each region of the spine are somewhat different in shape and size (see figure 1.1). The cervical vertebrae, for example, are smaller and flatter than those in the thoracic or lumbar region. Each of these bones is separated by an intervertebral disc above and below it.

INTERVERTEBRAL DISCS

The discs located between each vertebra function as shock absorbers *and* as joints. They absorb the stresses your spine experiences during daily activities, while allowing the vertebral bodies to move. The discs are made up of a strong outer ring of fibers called the **annulus fibrosis** and a soft center called the **nucleus pulposus**. The outer layer (annulus) helps keep the disc's inner layer (nucleus) intact. The strong fibers of the annulus also help connect one vertebra to the next. The nucleus of the disc has a high water content and a gel-like consistency.

FACET JOINTS

The facets connect the bony arches of the vertebral bodies. There are two **facet joints** between each pair of vertebrae, one on each side. Facet joints connect each vertebra with the next one, above and below, and allow the vertebral bodies to bend forward and backward, and to rotate, also providing stability. Similar to the other joints throughout your body, they are richly supplied with sensory nerve endings.

NEURAL FORAMEN

The neural foramen is the opening where the nerve roots exit the spine and travel to the rest of the body. There are two neural foramen, located between each pair of vertebrae, one on each side (figure 1.2). The foramen creates a protective passageway for the nerves to carry signals between the spinal cord and the rest of the body.

SPINAL LIGAMENTS

Ligaments are bands of fibrous tissue that connect bone to bone; in your back, they help stabilize the spinal column. The major spinal ligaments are the anterior longitudinal and posterior longitudinal ligaments, which run from the neck to the sacrum (top to bottom) in the front and back of the spinal column, keeping the vertebrae in place. Other, smaller ligaments extend between the spinal lamina

My Neck Hurts!

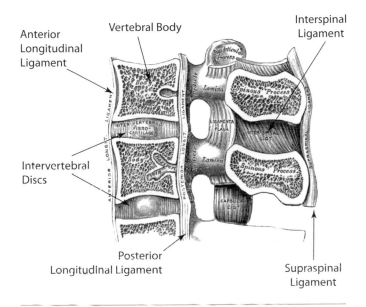

Anterior Longitudinal Ligament

Vertebral Body

Interspinal Ligament

Intervertebral Discs

Posterior Longitudinal Ligament

Supraspinal Ligament

FIGURE 1.5 Longitudinal cross-section of the spinal column and spinal ligaments. Adapted from figure 301 in *Henry Gray*, 20th ed., rev. and ed. Warren H. Lewis, Philadelphia: Lea and Febiger, 1918.

(ligamentum flavaum) and between the spinous processes (interspinal ligaments). The supraspinal ligament runs in the same direction as longitudinal ligaments along the back of the spinous processes (see figure 1.5).

MUSCLES OF THE NECK AND UPPER BACK

Muscles are commonly involved in chronic pain. Muscular pain can radiate from the origin and involve several areas; for example, your pain may be radiating from your neck into the back of your head (the occiput), across the shoulders, and into the upper back. One of the largest muscles extending over the neck and upper back is the trapezius. This muscle covers deeper muscles, which run across the lower neck,

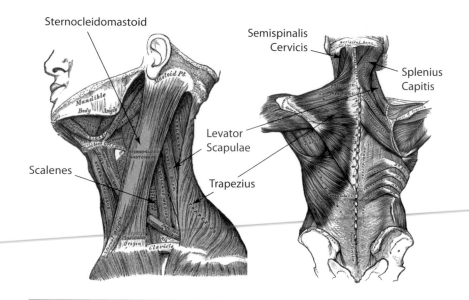

FIGURE 1.6   The muscles of the neck and upper back commonly involved in chronic neck pain. Adapted from figure 301 in *Henry Gray*, 20th ed., rev. and ed. Warren H. Lewis, Philadelphia: Lea and Febiger, 1918.

shoulders, and upper back. The levator scapulae runs between the scapula (shoulder blade) and the vertebrae of the neck to help raise the shoulder. Running parallel along the cervical spine are layers of muscle, including the semispinalis cervicis and splenius capitis. Backward movement (extension) and rotation of the neck are both facilitated by these muscles and other, smaller fibers that attach to the back of the skull. Muscles in the front and sides of the neck are less commonly involved with chronic pain. They include the sternocleidomastoid and scalene muscles, which rotate and side-bend the neck, respectively (see figure 1.6).

NOW THAT YOU ARE FAMILIAR with the anatomy of the cervical spine and its surrounding structures, it's time to examine why you are experiencing pain. The next chapter covers the most common medical conditions that contribute to chronic neck and upper back pain, from sprain and strain to disc disease and arthritis. The next chapter also describes diagnostic tests used to help identify the sources of your pain.

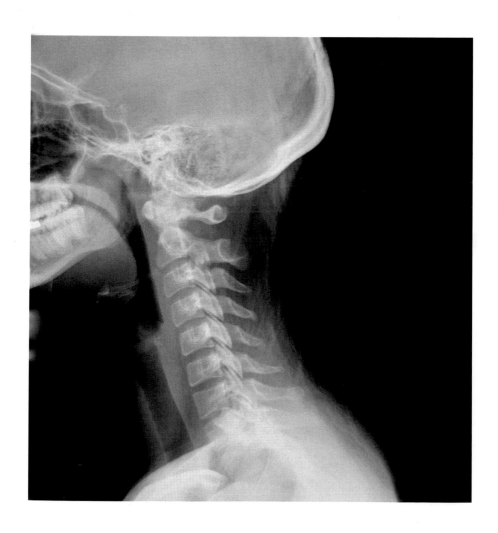

What's Causing Your Neck and Upper Back Pain?

Many factors can play a role in chronic neck and upper back pain. There is usually not a *single* cause but multiple abnormalities that together cause **symptoms**, including pain, stiffness, muscle spasm, and numbness or tingling. Although it is natural for you to want to compare notes with friends or family members, do so with caution, because two people can have similar symptoms but very different underlying pathology.

In addition to problems in the physical structures of

the neck, described in chapter 1, there are a host of other potential contributors to your pain, including age, gender, work environment, stress, anxiety level, past or current illnesses, physical activity, and even your psychological health. This is why your physician will ask you questions about aspects of your life that may seem unrelated to the purpose of your visit and why it is important for you to answer these questions thoroughly. The information you provide, along with what you and your doctor learn from examinations and diagnostic tests, will help identify the source of the problem and the best treatment options for you.

This chapter reviews the most common contributing factors in chronic neck and upper back pain. Becoming familiar with these factors will help you as you and your doctor investigate what is causing your pain. The less common, and sometimes serious, causes of pain need to be ruled out by your physician and are *not* addressed in this book. These include but are not limited to spinal infection, cancer, compression fractures, **Arnold Chiari malformation**, arachnoiditis, **discitis, scoliosis, torticollis, ankylosing spondylitis, systemic lupus erythematosus**, infectious meningitis, spinal instability, and congenital deformities.

PUTTING A NUMBER ON YOUR PAIN

An accurate and detailed history can help your doctor identify the most likely reasons for your pain and help him or her decide what type of testing may be needed. Think about what you want to tell your doctor before your visit and consider writing a list of symptoms so you don't forget anything important. Describe your pain in detail regarding the severity, quality, frequency, location, and any associated symptoms. Your doctor will find it helpful if you can answer most of the following questions at your appointment:

How bad or severe is the pain?
Can you describe the quality of your pain?

How often does the pain occur?

Where is the pain?

What makes the pain better or worse?

Are you having any symptoms in the arms?

Are there any associated symptoms with your pain?

How does your pain affect your ability to function physically, emotionally, and socially?

What was the situation and timing when the pain first started?

- **How bad or severe is the pain?**

  Pain is very subjective and therefore difficult to quantify. It can be defined as a sensory experience that is noxious or unpleasant, with both physical and emotional components. Your doctor needs to understand how bad your pain feels on different days and at different times. Your pain will wax and wane to some degree on a daily and even weekly basis, depending on your level of activity and your emotional state. For this reason, keeping a journal of simple notes recording your day-to-day experience of pain will be very helpful to your physician. Remember, you are intimately familiar with your pain and other symptoms; your doctor is not.

  Pain is typically rated on a numeric scale from 0 (no pain) to 10 (maximum, or worst pain possible). Figure 2.1 shows an example of this type of scale with the corresponding **Wong-Baker FACES Pain Rating Scale**, which was developed as a tool to help patients (including pediatric patients as young as age three) rate their pain for nurses and physicians. Even people who cannot read can understand the expressions on the faces. Do not underestimate or overestimate your pain level—an inaccurate estimation in either direction is counterproductive. To say that your pain is an 11 or outside the range of the scale does not help your physician understand your suffering. It may be helpful to report what a "10 out of 10" pain would be for you based on your prior experiences (kidney stones, childbirth). If you have not had such an experience, a

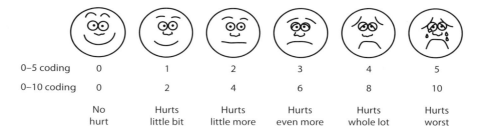

0–5 coding	0	1	2	3	4	5
0–10 coding	0	2	4	6	8	10
	No hurt	Hurts little bit	Hurts little more	Hurts even more	Hurts whole lot	Hurts worst

FIGURE 2.1   The Wong-Baker FACES Pain Rating Scale to help patients rate their pain for the nurses and physicians caring for them. From M. J. Hockenberry, D. Wilson, and M. L. Winkelstein, *Wong's Essentials of Pediatric Nursing*, 7th ed., St. Louis, 2005, p. 1259. Used with Permission. Copyright, Mosby.

"10 out of 10" could be described as the worst pain you can imagine, making it impossible to walk, talk, or move. I ask my patients to rate their pain range on this numeric scale by describing the minimal and maximal pain level as well as the average.

- Can you describe the quality of your pain?

  The quality of your pain may vary depending on your level of activity, the time of day, and your emotional state. Use terms such as sharp or shooting, nagging or achy, dull, throbbing or pulsating, steady, boring, squeezing or bandlike, or burning. Your notes will help you answer this question in a way that will be helpful to your doctor.

- How often does the pain occur?

  Is the pain present all the time, or is it only present on and off? Is it worse in the morning or later in the day, during or after work?

- Where is the pain?

  Does it start in the neck, upper back, or shoulders? Is it worse on one side or usually equal? Does it radiate into the head or into the arms?

- What makes the pain better or worse?

  Does sitting, bending, standing, walking, driving, or any specific activity at home or work affect the level or quality of your pain?

- Are you having any symptoms in the arms?
  Do you have any tingling, numbness, pain, or weakness in the arms?
- Are there any associated symptoms with your pain?
  Do you have restricted or reduced range of motion in the neck or shoulders? Do you have dizziness, headaches, nausea, fatigue, or problems with balance?
- How does your pain affect your ability to function physically, emotionally, and socially?
  Rate the effect of your pain on daily activities as follows:
  1 = There is no reduction in my normal activity.
  2 = The pain is disturbing and limits some of my normal activity, but bed rest is not necessary.
  3 = My normal daily activity has to be stopped, and bed rest may be necessary.
  4 = Bed rest is necessary.
  Does the pain keep you from falling or staying asleep? Do you feel tired in the morning or throughout the day because of pain? Does your pain make you feel sad, depressed, or anxious? Does your pain prevent you from attending social activities with friends or family? Does your pain affect your emotional or sexual relationship with your significant other? Is your ability to work or take care of your family affected?
- What was the situation and timing when the pain first started?
  Did any physical or emotional injury occur when the pain started? Has it been the same since the onset, or has it worsened recently? Did any injury occur at home, in public, or at work? Is there any litigation or compensation process involved?

SPRAIN AND STRAIN

Cervical sprains and strains involve an overstretching or tearing in the supporting tissues of the neck. A **sprain** results from injury to the *ligaments* and a **strain** from injury to the *muscles or muscle tendon*. Sprained or strained tissue becomes tender to the touch, and results in stiffness, swelling, and reduced range of motion in the neck. Other associated symptoms can include headache, dizziness, numbness, tingling, pain, or weakness in the arms.

Cervical sprains and strains typically occur together and are usually a result of one of two common causes: long-term or excessive physical activity or sudden trauma. These types of injuries frequently occur in people whose occupation requires excessive or repetitive use of their arms or awkward head positions, such as working on an assembly line, in auto repair, and even working in an office at a computer with poor ergonomics. Sudden trauma, such as an auto accident, fall, or sports injury, can also cause cervical sprains and strains.

Whiplash is a common cause of a sprain/strain injury. It is also the most common type of injury resulting from a motor vehicle accident. The force at impact causes sudden, excessive extension (backward motion) and then rapid flexion (forward motion) of the neck (figure 2.2). A more severe ligament injury can even cause instability of the spine. This can be detected in routine x-rays. Whiplash motion can also cause trauma to the facet joints. Other, more serious injuries to the vertebrae or intervertebral discs are possible but less likely.

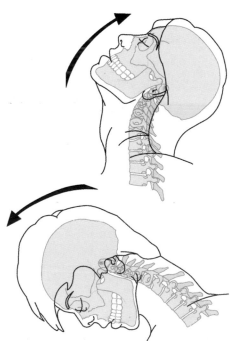

People usually report pain from whiplash shortly after an

FIGURE 2.2 Excessive cervical extension (*top*) and flexion (*bottom*) from a typical whiplash injury. © Fotosearch.

My Neck Hurts!

accident, but sometimes the pain doesn't begin until several days later. After the injury, the muscles surrounding the neck and head stiffen up. Over time, this stiffness may spread from the neck to the upper back muscles. Associated symptoms can occur, including headaches, dizziness, and arm pain or tingling.

Most of the time, your body heals from whiplash, with minimal treatment, over the course of several weeks. Treatment includes heat application, **nonsteroidal anti-inflammatory drugs** (**NSAIDs**, such as ibuprofen and naproxen) or **muscle relaxants** such as Flexeril, and **physical therapy.**

ARTHRITIS

Arthritis is inflammation and stiffness of a joint that may result in swelling and restricted motion. Arthritic disorders can complicate neck pain in many people.

Osteoarthritis is a degenerative joint disease that occurs in everyone as they age and tends to worsen over time. In fact, osteoarthritis occurs in more than half the population over age 50. That said, only some of these people suffer chronic pain. Osteoarthritis in the neck can be precipitated by an earlier trauma or degenerative disc disease. Increased friction, inflammation, and bone formation occur because of a mechanical breakdown in the cartilage lining the joint.

Over time, as a response to everyday stressors, our bones thicken to stabilize the spine. When excessive thickening occurs, the extra bone (called bone spurs, or **spondylosis**) can cause pain by compressing or irritating the exiting spinal nerve roots (**spinal stenosis**) or small nerves that supply the facet joints. Excessive bone formation can also extend into the spinal canal, compressing the spinal cord.

Several factors can increase the likelihood of developing severe osteoarthritis. Age is the primary and most predictable reason for osteoarthritis, often starting at around age 30. Work- or sports-related repetitive motion, or poor body mechanics, can set the stage for arthritis, particularly if you are overweight, because excess pounds place more stress on your joints. Genetic predisposition, poor circulation, or disease—such as diabetes—can also promote the onset and development of osteoarthritis.

Stiffness and pain are common features of osteoarthritis. These symptoms are typically at their worst first thing in the morning, lessening slightly as you become more active after rising. The pain can even awaken a person during the night. Many people with osteoarthritis experience a steady aching pain that is worsened by neck motion. Some people note that this pain becomes most acute during times of major weather changes. This is thought to be related to fluctuations in the barometric pressure and the heavier air that a low-pressure weather front brings.

Much less common types of arthritis include **rheumatoid arthritis**, psoriatic arthritis, gout, and ankylosing spondylitis.

DISC DISEASE

The number one question that people with neck or upper back pain ask their doctors is if a slipped disc is the cause of their pain. Although it is probably the most common concern, it is *not* the most common cause of neck pain. Surprisingly, many people with a disc problem do *not* experience neck pain.

When disc disease is the cause of pain, it typically results in compression or chemical irritation of a spinal nerve root. The fibrous outer shell of the disc (annulus fibrosis) can become torn or cracked by an acute injury or by chronic wear. The back (posterior) of the disc is most susceptible to this type of damage, which can also lead to herniation of the inner nucleus pulposus. Small tears in the disc can heal over time, but recurrent or large tears can result in a **bulging disc** (an intervertebral disc that extends beyond its normal boundary) or a **herniated disc** (when the inner nucleus pulposus extrudes through the outer annulus fibrosis; figure 2.3).

My Neck Hurts!

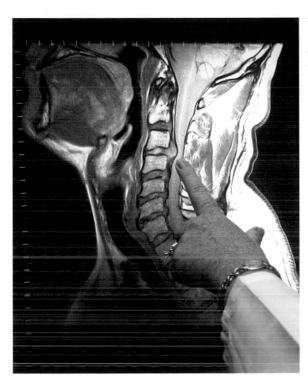

FIGURE 2.3   A herniated disc seen on an MRI scan. © 2006 Dean Hoch. Image from BigStockPhoto.com.

Large disc herniation in the cervical spine can cause narrowing of the central canal and, as a result, compression of the spinal cord. This compression can cause weakness and numbness not only in the arms but also in the legs. This is not an unusual scenario, yet most people—understandably—fail to attribute leg symptoms to neck problems. More commonly, a disc herniation causes narrowing of the spinal foramina, resulting in irritation or compression of a spinal nerve root. The location of the irritation or compression determines where symptoms are experienced in the body. These symptoms can include pain, numbness, tingling, or even weakness and can be present in the neck, upper trunk, or arms. For example, compression of the C8 nerve root (at the base of the neck) may result in numbness and tingling in the hand, while irritation of the C5 nerve root (at the middle of the neck) can cause symptoms in the shoulder region. Although some herniated discs require surgical repair, many patients respond to nonsurgical

What's Causing Your Neck and Upper Back Pain?   21 interventions, preventing or delaying a need for surgery. Nonsurgical options are described in the rest of this book.

FACET DISEASE

Pain caused by inflammation in or around the facet joints is called facet syndrome. This inflammation is typically a result of joint injury or arthritis. Facet joint pain is probably the most common cause of pain related to whiplash injury and occurs in a significant percentage of patients—26 to 65 percent—suffering from chronic neck pain. Symptoms of facet disease include tenderness to the touch over the facet joints, pain during neck movement that is worse on extension (tilting the head back) than on flexion (tilting the head forward), and pain that spreads into the shoulder or upper back regions. Neither x-rays nor MRI is particularly helpful in diagnosing facet disease because the images they provide can often appear normal even when facet disease is present. Facet disease is best diagnosed by diagnostic facet injections, which are discussed in depth in chapter 7.

MYOFASCIAL PAIN AND FIBROMYALGIA

Myofascial pain (MP) is a very common cause of chronic neck and upper back pain. This condition is frequently associated with a history of neck trauma, but it can occur as a result of chronic physical stressors such as a repetitive activity or overuse of the neck muscles and arms, excessive keyboarding, poor posture, and even emotional stress. Myofascial pain is commonly described as tight and achy, with stiffness, and it can be associated with limited ability to move the neck.

The hallmark of MP is regional pain involving multiple muscle groups and surrounding connective tissue in the neck and shoulders associated with trigger points. **Trigger points** can be consistently painful (active trigger points) or painful only when touched or pressed (latent trigger points). Trigger points in the neck cause localized pain as well as pain that spreads to other areas (**referred pain**), including the head, shoulders, and even the arms. Trigger points can correspond to known acupuncture points (discussed in chapter 8).

In most cases, trigger points meet the following clinical criteria:

- a hyper-irritable tender point that, when touched, feels like a taut ropelike band of muscle
- a "jump sign"—when pressure applied to the muscular area causes local and referred pain in a specific predictable pattern
- a twitch response, or temporary contraction of muscle fibers caused by sudden pressure or needling of the trigger point
- limited range of motion due to pain in the affected muscle

Areas with trigger points may have altered sensitivity and even abnormal sweating. Many individuals with MP report muscle weakness; this symptom is better described, however, as muscle fatigue. With fatigue, the muscles are less able to rebound after repetitive use. This condition is typically related to pain, whereas true muscle weakness (reduced strength unrelated to pain) can be a sign of nerve or muscle damage. No imaging studies or laboratory tests can diagnose MP, so diagnosis is made by a physician's clinical evaluation. Muscles typically involved in myofascial neck and upper back pain include the trapezius, supraspinatus, levator scapulae, rhomboids, and semispinalis (see figure 1.6).

Most people with any neck and upper back pain, regardless of the cause, have some element of myofascial pain. The diagnosis of MP is considered *primary* if no other structural abnormality is causing the muscular pain. If MP is the result of another underlying condition (such as a disc problem or facet disease), however, it is considered secondary. Whatever the underlying cause of the pain, most individuals with MP respond well to treatments such as physical therapy, medications such as nonsteroidal anti-inflammatory drugs, or muscle injections.

Fibromyalgia syndrome (FMS) is a chronic condition of unknown cause characterized by diffuse muscle pain and associated mood and sleep disturbances. The term *syndrome* is used to describe a constellation of clinical symptoms, in contrast to the term *disease*, which is used to describe medical conditions with established pathology, such as diabetes. As a syndrome, FMS is defined by specific symptoms and abnormalities that a physician can see on physical examination of a patient. The criteria for FMS were defined by the American College of Rheumatology in 1990 as follows:

1. widespread pain on both sides of the body and above and below the waistline for at least three months and
2. at least eleven of eighteen specific muscle **tender points**, on both sides of the body, including the neck, shoulders, back, hips, arms, and legs (Patients are not diffusely tender to touch all over the body.)

Individuals with FMS are typically most bothered by pain in their neck and shoulder regions. Other symptoms common in FMS can include

- poor quality sleep
- generalized fatigue
- headaches
- stiff joints
- depression, anxiety
- irritable bowl and bladder
- restless leg syndrome (RLS)
- cognitive and memory problems
- tingling in the extremities

Fibromyalgia syndrome is more common in women than in men and is believed to affect 2 to 4 percent of the American population. The

TABLE 2.1
Differences between trigger points typical in myofascial pain and tender points typical in fibromyalgia pain

	Trigger points	Tender points
Pain quality	Local tenderness, taut band, local twitch response, jump sign	Local tenderness
Number of points	Single or multiple points	Multiple points
Location	Can occur in any skeletal muscle	Occurs in specific locations on both sides of the body
Pain referral	Touch may cause a specific referred pain pattern	Touch does not cause referred pain but often causes an increase in pain sensitivity over the entire body

condition is chronic, but periods of remission are not uncommon. No current laboratory studies or x-rays can diagnose fibromyalgia, but a routine blood draw can help rule out more serious conditions, such as lupus erythematosus or rheumatoid arthritis, that can mimic FMS.

It can be difficult to distinguish between trigger points seen in MP and tender points present in FMS. Although the experience of pain is described similarly for both, making an accurate differentiation between trigger and tender points is essential, because MP and FMS are different diagnoses requiring different treatment. Diagnosis can be complicated when a person has both trigger and tender points. The qualitative differences between trigger and tender points are summarized in table 2.1.

RADICULOPATHY AND NEURALGIA

Radiculopathy is disease of a spinal nerve root. Typically, this disorder results from the compression or physical irritation of a spinal nerve root as it exits the neural foramen. The foraminal space can become narrowed by a disc herniation or by vertebral bone thickening (spurs), causing compression. Or the fluids ordinarily contained within a disc may leak out because of a tear, causing irritation and inflammation in a nearby nerve root. Less commonly, diseases such as shingles or diabetes similarly affect the spinal nerve roots by inflaming them. Any one of the eight cervical nerve roots can be involved in a radiculopathy, but the sixth and seventh nerves are the most commonly affected. Cervical radiculopathy can cause not only neck pain but also pain, numbness, and weakness down one or both arms.

Occipital neuralgia is a disorder commonly associated with chronic neck pain that is caused by irritation, compression,

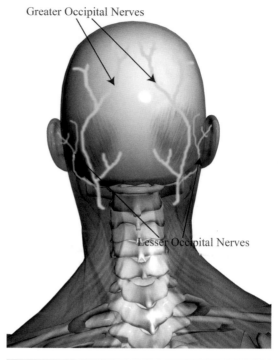

FIGURE 2.4   Distribution of the greater and lesser branches of the occipital nerves. © 2005 Patrick Hermans. Image adapted from BigStockPhoto.com.

or injury to an occipital nerve. There are several occipital nerves on each side of the base of the skull (occiput). These nerves originate from the second and third cervical nerve roots, which divide into a greater, lesser, and third branch (figure 2.4). Individuals with occipital neuralgia typically experience pain that starts at the nape of the neck. The pain is often described as throbbing and aching, commonly radiating into the back, side of the head, or both.

Less commonly, pain can radiate from the occiput to the eye or ear regions. Persons may also experience abnormal sensations in the back of the head, such as tingling, burning, or sharp shooting pain. Occipital neuralgia can be triggered by physical or emotional stress, trauma, or repeated contraction of the muscles of the neck. Headache syndromes, such as migraines or tension headaches, can be triggered by occipital neuralgia.

SPONDYLOLISTHESIS AND SPONDYLOLYSIS

Spondylolisthesis is a slipping of one vertebra over another. The most common cause of such slippage is **spondylolysis**, or a crack in the posterior portion of the vertebra that connects the spinous process to the facet joint. This defect can occur on one or both sides of the vertebra, and it is typically a result of chronic repetitive motion or trauma such as that experienced by professional athletes or industrial workers. Although spondylolisthesis usually occurs in the lower back, it can occur in the neck, especially in people who wear heavy head gear while working, such as welders.

PSYCHOSOCIAL FACTORS OF PAIN

Pain clearly has an emotional component to it, causing feelings of moodiness, depression, anxiety, helplessness, hopelessness, and even anger. It is not uncommon for my patients to tell me that they never felt depressed until they developed a chronic pain syndrome. Since pain can limit a person's enjoyment of simple things and decrease his or her ability to perform daily activities, depressed feelings are very likely to occur even in people who have never experienced depression. People with underlying psychiatric conditions may be more prone to develop a chronic pain state because they may be more sensitive to any abnormal sensation in their body. A cycle of pain causing depression and anxiety and depression and anxiety worsening pain can develop and be difficult to break.

Some trendy writers, as well as some physicians, have popularized the notion that almost all neck and back pain is caused by anxiety, depression, or repressed emotions. This extreme position is as incorrect and unhelpful as the opposite claim—that pain is entirely a result of physical injury or disease. Very few individuals experience pain that is purely psychological or purely physical in origin. The vast majority of patients with chronic neck and upper back pain have a physical basis for pain *and* experience the psychological consequences of that pain.

Together, pain and its accompanying emotions—anxious anticipation of pain and grief from loss of normal functioning—influence a person's social and family relationships. It is inadequate to simply state that there is a mind-body connection. There is a *reciprocal* mind-body relationship. Your physical health, especially any pain you are experiencing, affects your emotional and psychological health and overall feeling of well-being. No medical treatment plan is complete without a mental health plan that addresses the psychological impact of chronic pain.

In over ten years of treating patients with chronic neck and upper back pain, I have found that people who fail to experience any significant reduction in pain with multiple treatments usually have something going on in their lives that prevents them from following the recommended treatment plan or, more often, refuse to address the psychological issues that are perpetuating their cycle of pain. While most Americans appear to feel no stigma seeking care from a **neurologist** or physical therapist, many refuse to work with a pain counselor or a psychiatrist to develop a complementary mental health plan. Indeed, when I recommend a counselor or psychiatrist, many of my patients respond, "But I'm not crazy!"

Whatever the causes of your chronic neck and upper back pain, it can best be treated by a comprehensive plan that addresses physical *and* psychological causes and effects. Even the most psychologically well-adjusted individual will experience emotional consequences with extended periods of pain. You should feel no stigma as you smartly take advantage of every resource available when dealing with chronic pain.

People who are predisposed to anxiety or prolonged sadness but who have never developed a psychological disorder are likely to find that pain intensifies problems that have been manageable in the past. And people with significant mental health problems prior to developing chronic pain (as well as those with unusually high social stressors such as poverty, divorce, or a history of sexual abuse) may find that the entrance of chronic pain into their lives creates a nearly insurmountable obstacle to improvement in symptoms. When developing a treatment plan with your doctor, you need to include a way to address the mental and emotional components of your situation. To ignore the psychological consequences of pain is to dramatically reduce the likelihood of recovery.

DIAGNOSTIC TESTING

Your doctor will use diagnostic tests to aid in the evaluation of your chronic neck pain. Each test is designed to look for specific types of abnormalities in the anatomy or function of the cervical spine, muscles, ligaments, and nerves in and around the neck. The appropriate tests to be ordered will be determined by your medical history, a physical examination, and the clinical suspicions of your doctor. For example, if you suffered trauma to the neck in a motor vehicle accident, the emergency room doctor would order an x-ray to rule out a spinal fracture. If your neck pain is chronic, or you experience symptoms that extend into your arms, your doctor may order an MRI scan or an **electromyograph (EMG)** to rule out an abnormality in the intervertebral discs or spinal nerves.

X-ray (radiography) is the most commonly performed diagnostic test for patients with neck pain. X-rays expose the tissues to a form of electromagnetic radiation to create an anatomical image called a radiograph. The bones of the neck are best visualized with this technique when looking for fractures or other changes to the bones. Soft tissues such as muscles, intervertebral discs, and ligaments are not seen well with x-ray.

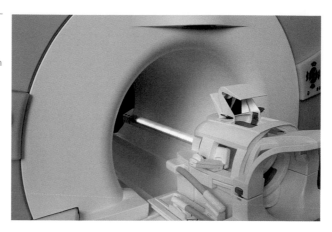

FIGURE 2.5 An MRI scanner. © 2006 Norman Chan. Image from BigStockPhoto.com.

Computer tomography (CT, commonly called a cat scan or c-t scan) also uses x-rays but with the aid of a computer for improved images. A series of cross-section images, or slices, are obtained in 5- to 10-millimeter increments, producing high-quality pictures of the region studied. The bones are seen better than in standard x-ray. When dye is injected through a spinal tap, the test is called **myelography**. When the dye enters the cerebrospinal fluid, the intervertebral discs, spinal canal, and neural foramina can also be visualized well.

Magnetic resonance imaging (MRI), unlike an x-ray, does not expose the body to any radiation (figure 2.5). Instead, it uses the property of the body's atoms to form images that differentiate between bone, disc, muscle, and fat. As with CT scans, high-quality slices are produced with this technique. Soft tissues such as intervertebral discs and muscles are seen very well, which is why MRIs are more frequently ordered than CTs to evaluate possible disc pathology. Patients with pacemakers, defibrillators, and some other implantable devices with metal *cannot* have an MRI.

Electromyography with **nerve conduction studies (NCS)** is used to evaluate the health of the spinal nerves that come out of the neck and the nerves in the arms and hands. This test helps determine if there is a compressed or pinched spinal nerve (radiculopathy). It can also assess the general health of the nerves and test for compression of a **peripheral nerve** in the arm or hand, as occurs in carpal tunnel syndrome. This test is very useful in determining the location of a **pinched nerve**, which is important, because different locations of compression can produce similar symptoms, such as numbness, tingling, or pain in an arm or a hand.

The nerve conduction portion of the test is performed first. Wires are attached to the skin of the symptomatic arm with electrodes (metal disks or stickers). An electrical current is sent along the nerve with a device that touches the skin. This impulse is not painful and will not harm the nerve, but it is surprising. A muscle may twitch, which is a normal response. Electromyography is then performed. A fine needle is inserted into muscles of the symptomatic arm. The needle may need to be moved around to sample different regions of the muscle. Muscle cramping, pain, or pressure may be experienced as the muscle is contracted. No electrical impulse is given in this portion of the test.

MAKING A MEDICAL DIAGNOSIS is a bit like solving a mystery. You can provide your physician with clues by keeping a simple journal with details that answer the questions in the first section of this chapter. Once your doctor has identified the cause of your pain and made a diagnosis, together you can begin to develop the best treatment plan for you.

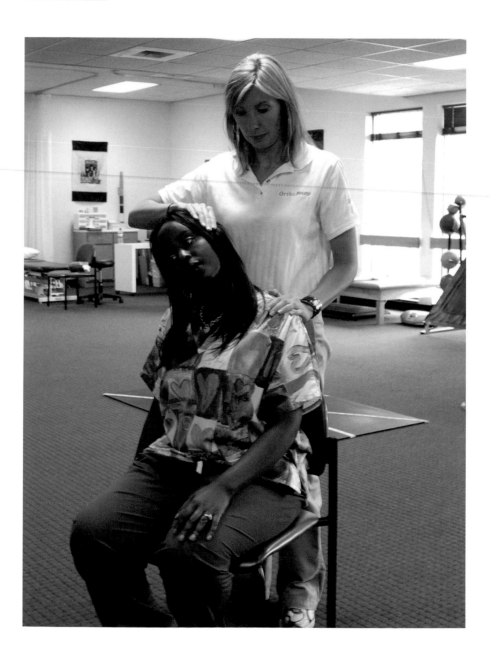

How Physical Therapy
Can Help

Physical therapy is one of the most frequently pre-scribed treatments for chronic neck pain. In most states, access to physical therapy does not require a prescription, and you may seek treatment on your own. A referral to a physical therapist from your physician, however, which includes an accurate diagnosis and the results of pertinent diagnostic testing, is the best way to begin. And for health insurance reimbursement, a pre-scription from your physician may be required.

Before you make a physical therapy appointment, ask

if the therapist has experience treating chronic neck and upper back pain, and if he or she has any manual therapy skills (more about that later in this chapter and in chapter 5). The quality of your experience will be greatly influenced by the therapist's training and expertise, as well as by the treatment **modalities** ordered by your physician. The effects of your physical therapy may also vary as you and the therapist progress through different stages of your treatment.

Treatment begins with a comprehensive evaluation by the physical therapist, who will take a history to evaluate the level, quality, and location of your pain. He or she will also assess your functional limitations, strength, range of motion, posture, and balance. Based on the results of this assessment, the physical therapist will discuss the findings with you and develop a treatment plan. The therapist should also be in communication with the referring physician as well as other practitioners involved in your care so that all providers are informed of and in agreement with the treatment plan.

The goals of your treatment should be reasonable and achievable. Most physical therapy goals are based on reducing pain and increasing functional performance and range of motion for the neck and shoulder region—in other words, getting you back to preinjury or predisability activities (or as close to that as possible). When you begin physical therapy, keep these two facts in mind: improvement will not happen overnight, and your commitment to attend all sessions regularly *and* to perform home exercises and stretches as instructed is essential for success.

Physical therapy involves exercise, but often it also involves the use of modalities. Modalities are treatments used as part of a physical therapy session, including heat, cold, ultrasound, electrical stimulation, and traction. These treatments are used to reduce pain before or after stretching and other exercise and to maximize the effect of the therapy. Modalities used in physical therapy are described later in this chapter.

■ Getting Back in the Water

Jerry was a 62-year-old retired investment banker when he first sought help for his chronic neck pain. He underwent a cervical fusion for spinal stenosis, and even though the surgery at first eliminated much of his neck pain, it left him with limited range of motion in the cervical spine as well as intermittent dizziness. "My neck was always tight, and I had spasms of pain. My range of motion was decreased since the surgery, making it hard to do things like back up my car."

Over time, his neck and upper back pain got worse and included his left arm and shoulder. The pain was most pronounced after his daily swim (his favorite form of exercise) at the local Y. He liked to swim freestyle, turning his head to the left, but the pain and limited mobility was making that almost impossible. "Swimming, which I had enjoyed since high school, seemed to exacerbate the problem. My muscles would feel completely tight, like a wall. It was constantly annoying."

His primary care physician referred him to a physical therapist for evaluation and treatment. During his initial exam, the therapist noted limited motion in both the cervical and thoracic spine, as well as postural changes that included a "forward head" and increase in thoracic kyphosis (increased, exaggerated curve in spine). Jerry explained that he had always prided himself on staying trim and in shape and was frustrated at having to give up most of his exercise activities due to pain and lack of mobility. Taking into account his love of exercise and his physical condition, the therapist recommended a combination of physical therapy treatments.

Manual therapy, including **muscle energy,** scapular mobilization, **myofascial release,** and soft tissue massage was performed, along with stretching and postural exercises. He also received heat and electric stimulation treatments.

Jerry was diligent about his therapy and after sixteen sessions had achieved a marked improvement in cervical range of motion, a significant decrease in pain, and—most satisfying to Jerry—the ability to return to the pool for his daily swim.

EXERCISE

There are three different forms of exercise: stretching, strengthening, and aerobic, or cardiovascular conditioning. An appropriate exercise program can maintain the functional capacity of your musculoskeletal system with little effort. It is important that you understand and commit to performing the appropriate exercise program. Your therapist will prescribe a program specifically for your pain profile and current level of strength and mobility. He or she will probably provide take-home sheets illustrating your exercises, but bring this book with you when you meet. By looking at the illustrations together, you can be certain that you understand the therapist's instructions, and your therapist can tell you which exercises might help you and which you should avoid.

Stretching

Stretching exercises, or flexibility exercises, are designed to increase mobility and range of motion and to decrease tightness or spasm. Stretching can be performed in the *static* or *dynamic* mode. Neither type of stretching should cause significant pain or other symptoms, such as abnormal sensations in the arms, although mild discomfort is acceptable.

- Static stretches are performed by holding a position that lengthens the muscle and connective tissue. They should be done carefully, with a maximum hold time of 30 seconds.
- Dynamic stretches are more active and should be performed within your available range of motion two to three times a day, in 10 to 20 repetitions. Either may be preceded by heat or an aerobic (warm-up) activity.

The following exercises are examples of a typical exercise regimen for neck and upper back pain (see figures 3.1–3.8). Your physical therapist will guide you through practice stretches and strengthening exercises that are best for you; you should perform them regularly at home. These exercises can also be used during breaks from your daily activities to promote relaxation and proper posture. *Check with your physician or physical therapist before performing any of these stretches or exercises on your own.*

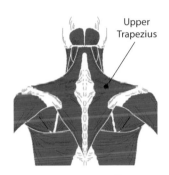

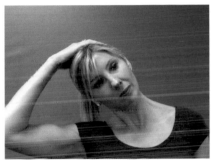

FIGURE 3.1   Upper trapezius stretch: Tilt your head away from the tight side. Drawing © 2009 Wolters Kluwer Health | Lippincott Williams and Wilkins.

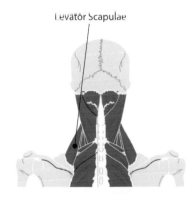

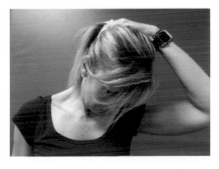

FIGURE 3.2   Levator stretch: Pull your head down and rotate it away from the tight side. Drawing © 2009 Wolters Kluwer Health | Lippincott Williams and Wilkins.

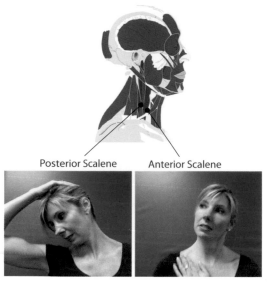

FIGURE 3.3 Posterior scalene stretch: Tilt your head and rotate your neck away from the tight side. Anterior scalene stretch: Pull down on your collarbone, tuck your chin, and look over your shoulder. Drawing © 2009 Wolters Kluwer Health | Lippincott Williams and Wilkins.

Posterior Scalene   Anterior Scalene

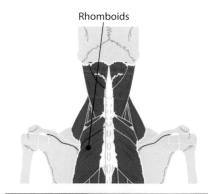

Rhomboids

FIGURE 3.4 Rhomboid stretch: Pull your arm across your chest, away from the tight side. Drawing © 2009 Wolters Kluwer Health | Lippincott Williams and Wilkins.

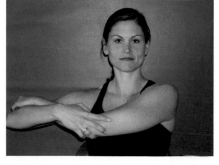

My Neck Hurts!

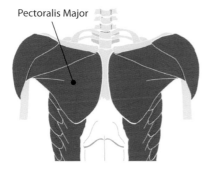

Pectoralis Major

FIGURE 3.5 Pectoralis major stretch: Face a corner or doorway with arms raised and push your chest forward. Drawing © 2009 Wolters Kluwer Health I Lippincott Williams and Wilkins.

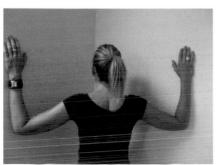

Pectoralis Minor

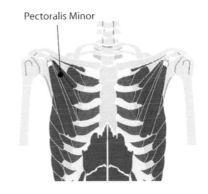

FIGURE 3.6 Pectoralis minor stretch: Place your hand flat on the wall with an out-stretched arm and turn away from the tight pectoralis. Drawing © 2009 Wolters Kluwer Health I Lippincott Williams and Wilkins.

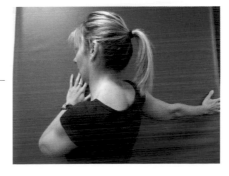

How Physical Therapy Can Help

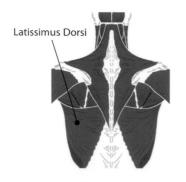

Latissimus Dorsi

FIGURE 3.7   Latissimus dorsi stretch: Kneel with elbows on a chair, forearms pointed upward, then drop your upper back down, with extended arms. Drawing © 2009 Wolters Kluwer Health | Lippincott Williams and Wilkins.

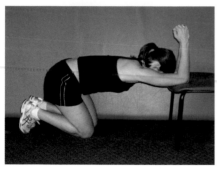

FIGURE 3.8   Latissimus dorsi stretch: Kneel in prayer position and drop your upper back down, forehead to the floor, arms stretched in front of you.

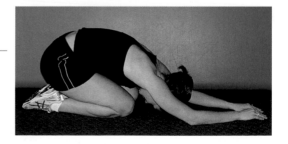

My Neck Hurts!

Strengthening

Strengthening exercises for cervical (neck) and scapular (shoulder blade) stabilization are designed to improve the strength of the postural muscles. These exercises should be performed at least three times per week.

The following exercises are commonly prescribed to strengthen cervical and scapular musculature, including the cervical flexors and extensors, lower trapezius, serratus anterior, rhomboids, and shoulder elevators (figures 3.9–3.13). Check with your physician or physical therapist before performing any of these exercises on your own.

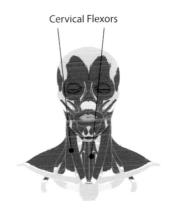

Cervical Flexors

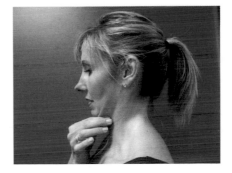

FIGURE 3.9   Cervical flexion strengthening (chin tucks): Tuck in chin to chest, activating deep neck flexors. Hold 6 seconds. Do not allow movement of neck. Perform 5 to 10 repetitions. Drawing © 2009 Wolters Kluwer Health | Lippincott Williams and Wilkins.

Cervical Extensors

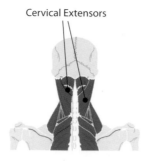

FIGURE 3.10 Isometric cervical extension: Place hands behind head and turn head slightly, pushing head backward into hands. Hold 6 seconds, not allowing movement of neck, 5 to 10 times. Drawing © 2009 Wolters Kluwer Health | Lippincott Williams and Wilkins.

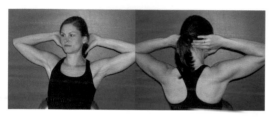

Lower Trapezius   Serratus Anterior

FIGURE 3.11 Lower trapezius and serratus anterior strengthening: In (A) a standing position and in (B) a kneeling prayer position, squeeze the shoulder blades together (scapular retraction) and back to a V shape. Hold 6 seconds. Perform 10 repetitions. Drawing © 2009 Wolters Kluwer Health | Lippincott Williams and Wilkins.

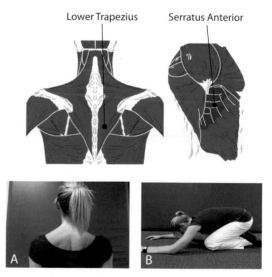

A   B

My Neck Hurts!

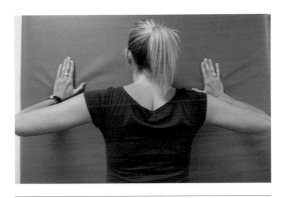

FIGURE 3.12   Lower trapezius and serratus anterior strengthening: Perform a wall push-up by squeezing the shoulder blades together and dropping into the wall. Finish by extending arms. Perform up to 30 repetitions.

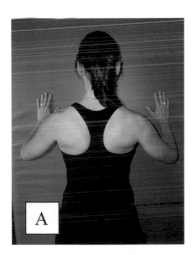
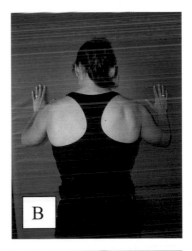

FIGURE 3.13   Rhomboids: (A) Perform a wall press by squeezing the shoulder blades together with forearms on the wall. (B) Drop head down and pull shoulder blades apart. Hold 5 to 10 seconds each direction. Perform 10 repetitions.

If your abdominal musculature (figure 3.14) is weak or you have lower back pain, it may be important to include lower quadrant exercises in your routine, because poor lower back posture can worsen neck strain. Be sure to ask your therapist to evaluate this area as well. The following are examples of exercises prescribed to strengthen lower back and "core" abdominal muscles (figures 3.15 and 3.16).

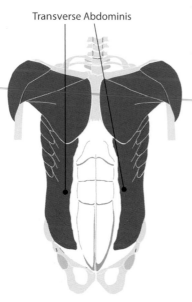

Transverse Abdominis

FIGURE 3.14   Transverse abdominis muscles. © 2009 Wolters Kluwer Health | Lippincott Williams and Wilkins.

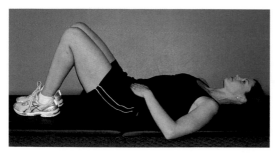

FIGURE 3.15   Isometric abdominal contraction: Lying on your back, with knees bent, draw in your lower abdominal muscles by tightening your stomach below the navel. Exhale or cough to help find them. Hold for 6 seconds 10 times. Try placing a pillow between your legs if your back hurts while performing this exercise.

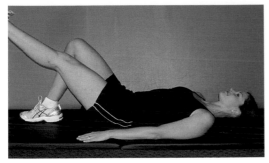

FIGURE 3.16 Single leg raise: Lying on your back, with knees bent, hold your belly tight and gradually raise and straighten one leg, keeping the other leg bent at the knee. Do not let the pelvis rock. Begin with 10 repetitions and increase as you are able for up to 2 minutes. Repeat the same exercise with the other leg.

Aerobic

Aerobic exercise is cardiovascular conditioning. During any aerobic exercise, your heart's beats per minute will increase, your breathing will become more exaggerated, and you will perspire. This type of exercise is important in stimulating endorphin levels and reducing pain generators. Aerobic exercise is also instrumental in weight loss, which is important for decreasing strain on the postural musculature. Aerobic exercise includes walking, jogging, in-line skating, biking, swimming, tennis, and the use of any low-impact equipment at your local health club such as an elliptical machine or stationary bike (see examples in figures 3.17 and 3.18). Low-impact exercises are preferable to high-impact exercises such as jogging because they provide cardio-vascular conditioning without jarring the body, which can make neck pain worse. Aerobic activity should be performed three to four times a week for 20- to 40-minute sessions. The following aerobic exercises can help to tone the upper back and neck. Check with your physician or physical therapist before performing any of these exercises on your own.

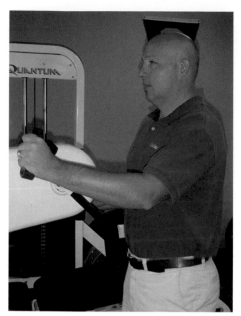

FIGURE 3.17 Demonstration of an upper body ergometer, used to develop arm strength and for low-impact aerobic exercise.

FIGURE 3.18 Riding a stationary bicycle is a great aerobic exercise that keeps the spine stabilized. Some bicycles are equipped with arm levers for upper arm conditioning. © 2005 Pavel Losevsky. Image from BigStockPhoto.com.

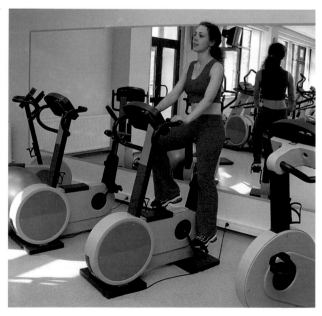

My Neck Hurts!

BAND AND BODY BALL THERAPY

When you have mastered the basic exercises, adding resistance with elastic bands or tubing is optimal. Elastic bands or tubing provide variable resistance throughout the range of motion. Check with your physician or physical therapist before performing any of the following exercises on your own (figures 3.19–3.22).

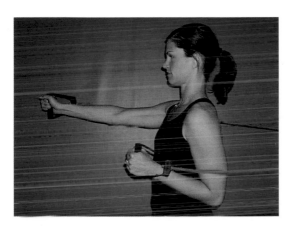

FIGURE 3.19 Single arm tubing punches: Attach bands to a stationary object or close them in a door frame. Alternate arms, pushing the band forward 10 to 30 times with each arm.

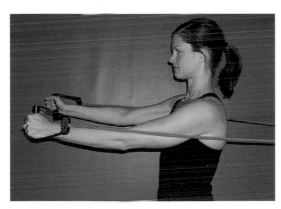

FIGURE 3.20 Double arm tubing punches: Attach bands to a stationary object or close in a door frame. Push both bands forward at the same time 10 to 30 times.

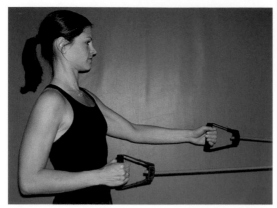

FIGURE 3.21 Single arm tubing rows: Face the bands and pinch your shoulder blades together. Alternate pulling the bands toward yourself 10 to 30 times on each arm.

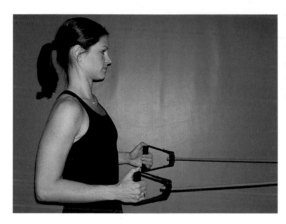

FIGURE 3.22 Double arm tubing rows: Face the bands and pinch your shoulder blades together. Pull both bands toward yourself 10 to 30 times.

Because therapy balls provide an unstable surface on which to exercise, they help develop core postural muscles and add interest and challenge to your exercise routine. Make sure your ball is the appropriate size for your frame and that it is inflated to the correct level. Check with your physician or physical therapist before performing any of the following exercises on your own (figures 3.23–3.27).

My Neck Hurts!

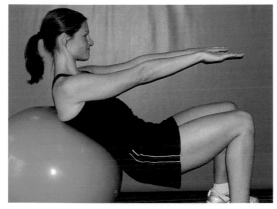

FIGURE 3.23   Squat and rock: Lean back on the ball and tuck in your chin, arms stretched out straight in front of you. Allow your bottom to sink to the floor and then return. Perform 10 to 30 repetitions.

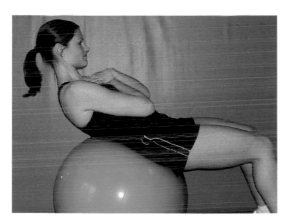

FIGURE 3.24   Sit backs: Tuck in your chin and roll back on the ball. Do not arch your back. If this causes back pain, reposition and try again. Performed correctly, this exercise should not cause pain. Perform 10 to 30 repetitions.

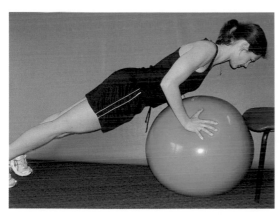

FIGURE 3.25   Floor push-ups: (This is an advanced exercise.) Stabilize the ball against the wall or a chair. Perform a push-up 10 to 30 times.

How Physical Therapy Can Help

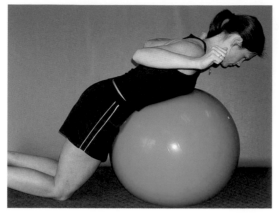

FIGURE 3.26   Over-ball W: Lie over ball and make a W with your shoulder blades by holding your shoulders down and back, pushing back with your elbows. Hold for 6 seconds 10 to 20 times.

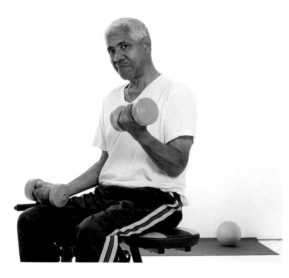

FIGURE 3.27   Hand weights can be used seated or standing. © 2008 Rob Marmion. Image from BigStockPhoto.com.

Free weights are exercise weights you hold in your hands to work a particular muscle group, in contrast to using a weight machine, where the weights are a "fixed" part of the machine and can be used only in a particular manner. Free weights provide resistance to your muscles through both pulling and pushing motions. Begin with a low weight (hand weights begin in sizes as low as one pound) that is comfortable to use without straining. You should be able to perform 2 to 3 sets of 10 repetitions comfortably before you begin to increase the weight gradu-

My Neck Hurts!

ally. The pictures that follow illustrate several exercises to strengthen the upper body using dumbbells while sitting on a therapy ball (see

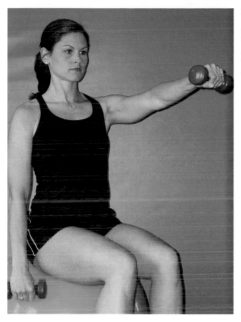

figures 3.28–3.31). Check with your physician or physical therapist before performing any of these exercises on your own.

FIGURE 3.28   Shoulder flexion: Raise your arm straight out and then lower it. Perform 2 to 3 sets of 10 repetitions with each arm.

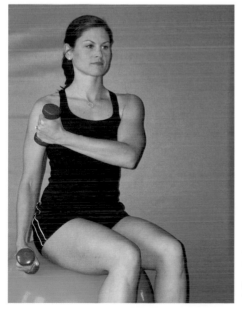

FIGURE 3.29   Upper cuts: Lift your arm across your chest. Perform 2 to 3 sets of 10 repetitions with each arm.

How Physical Therapy Can Help

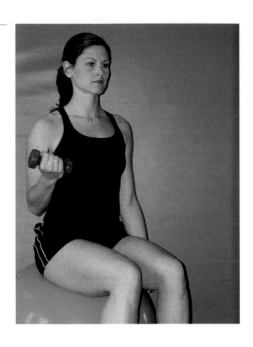

FIGURE 3.30 Biceps curls: Flex your elbow, and then straighten one arm at a time. Perform 2 to 3 sets of 10 repetitions.

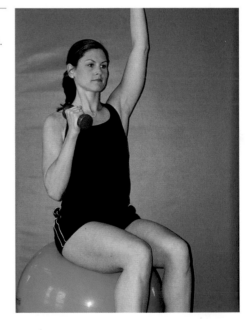

FIGURE 3.31 Overhead press: Raise each arm above your head one at a time. Perform 2 to 3 sets of 10 repetitions.

Under the instruction of your therapist, many other exercises can be performed using small hand-held weights (dumbbells) or large bar weights (barbells), depending on your general health and level of fitness. The preceding exercises are a good start for most patients.

My Neck Hurts!

■ Getting Physical

Kendall was a healthy 27-year-old when she gave birth to her second child. It was a joyful occasion, but the strain of pushing during labor resulted in a nerve injury (spontaneous brachial plexopathy, an inflammation of nerves in the underarm), leaving her with pain in her neck and left shoulder.

Soon after, she tried physical therapy and found that it helped, but as a busy mom, she didn't stay with it. That was seventeen years ago, and since then, although her symptoms have improved, she continues to have persistent aching in her left shoulder blade and upper back. The pain worsens if she lies on her left shoulder while sleeping. She also has some tingling in her left hand when her arm is in certain positions, and she frequently experiences weakness in her left arm and shoulder. Despite these problems, x-rays of her neck and an electromyography (EMG) of the left arm have not revealed anything abnormal.

By age 45, with a demanding job as a tax analyst, she was tired of dealing with the pain and decided it was time to try physical therapy again. "With my kids grown, I had more time to focus on my health."

Her initial PT treatment included manipulation of the upper back and shoulder region, a series of stretching and flexibility exercises, and scapular stabilization exercises. Her sessions, which also included intermittent ice application and electrical stimulation, were scheduled two to three times a week for six weeks.

By the end of Kendall's treatment she had a significant decrease in pain along with increased strength and postural stability. This led to an improved ability to perform her duties at work and activities at home. After completing six weeks of physical therapy, she now continues a regular routine of exercises and stretches at home. "I still experience some pain when lying on my shoulder at night, but overall my symptoms are mild and manageable during the day."

AQUATHERAPY

Exercising in water is an excellent way to strengthen the entire body with minimal impact on the joints. Standing in water that reaches between the navel and underarms, a person weighs only one-tenth of his or her dry-land body weight. Resistance exercises can be performed against the water alone or with the use of paddles, kickboards, fins, or water bottles. Moving your hips and shoulders through all planes of motion will strengthen the arms and legs as well as the trunk musculature. Check with your physician or physical therapist before performing any of the following exercises on your own (figure 3.32–3.42).

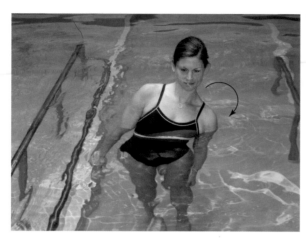

FIGURE 3.32   Side bends: Reach your arm to the knee, bending the upper body sideways at the waist. Perform 10 to 20 repetitions on each side.

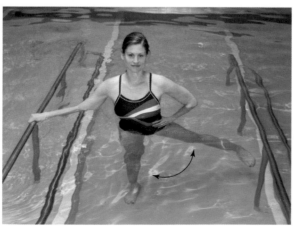

FIGURE 3.33   Side leg lifts: Stand on one leg and extend the other leg at the hip to the side. Perform 10 to 20 repetitions on each side.

My Neck Hurts!

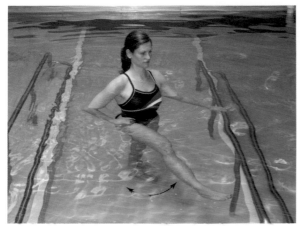

FIGURE 3.34 Forward leg lifts: Stand on one leg and extend the other leg at the hip to the front. Perform 10 to 20 repetitions on each leg.

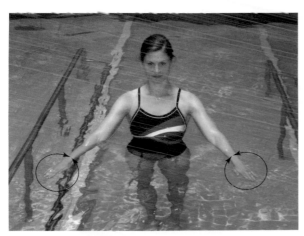

FIGURE 3.35 Arm circles: Move both arms in a clockwise and then counterclockwise motion at the same time. Perform 10 to 20 repetitions.

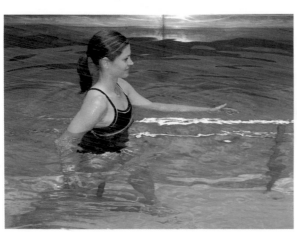

FIGURE 3.36 Walking: Forward, backward, and side step. Begin with 2 to 3 laps and increase to 10 as tolerated over time.

How Physical Therapy Can Help

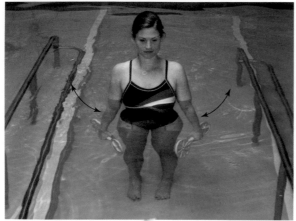

FIGURE 3.37 Side arm reaches: Sit or stand. Raise your arms to the side and lower. Keep your arms in the water. Perform 10 to 20 repetitions. If desired, this exercise, as well as the four that follow, can be performed with paddles, as seen here, to add more resistance.

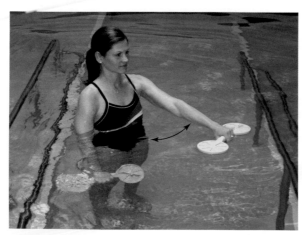

FIGURE 3.38 Forward arm reaches: Sit or stand. Raise your arms in front of you and then lower them. Keep your arms in the water. Perform 10 to 20 repetitions.

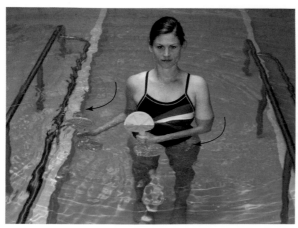

FIGURE 3.39 Arm rotation: Sit or stand. Push your arms right and then left with your elbows bent, together or apart. Keep your arms in the water. Perform 10 to 20 repetitions.

My Neck Hurts!

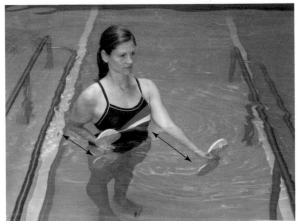

FIGURE 3.40 Punches: Sit or stand. Push your arm forward and then pull them back, pushing the other arm forward. Keep your arms in the water. Perform 10 to 20 on each arm.

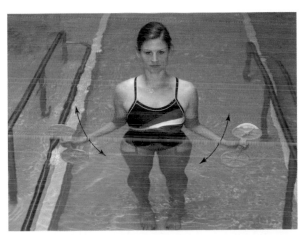

FIGURE 3.41 Butterflies: Sit or stand. Pull arms together in front of you and then apart. Keep your arms in the water. Perform 10 to 20 repetitions.

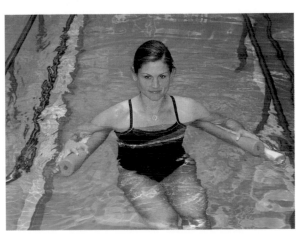

FIGURE 3.42 Unloading: Using Styrofoam "noodles," or tubes, or wearing an aqua vest to support you in the water provides relief to the lower back and is a great way to perform aerobic exercises that mimic jogging, bicycling, or marching. Stretching can also be performed in the water, usually after a land-based warm-up.

How Physical Therapy Can Help

The ideal temperature for the water is between 84 and 86 degrees Fahrenheit. People with arthritis may prefer warmer water, up to 90 degrees. Higher temperatures should not be used if you are pregnant.

ERGONOMICS AND POSTURE

Practicing good posture is critical in managing chronic neck or upper back pain (figure 3.43). Slumping over your computer, lying on your back with your head propped up on several pillows while you watch television, or reading with your head down on an airplane are all examples of bad posture and can make your pain worse. Correcting your posture is simple. Your pelvis naturally wants to shift forward. Sitting with your feet flat on the floor, rock your pelvis back and forth finding the midpoint, or neutral position. From here, gently draw your shoulders down and back to an imaginary V shape just between the shoulder blades. Slightly tuck your chin and think about a string coming out of the top of your head, gently pulling the head upward. Hold this position for 5 to 10 seconds and repeat five times every 30 to 60 minutes while you are performing a static activity, such as working at a computer.

If you wake up with a stiff neck, your sleep position may be aggravating your condition. Sleeping on your back with your head on a flat pillow made of down or buckwheat is ideal because it will keep your

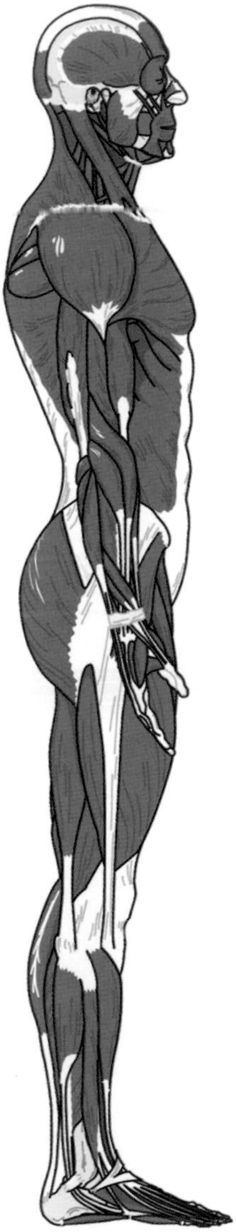

FIGURE 3.43   Proper posture positions the head so that the ears line up with the shoulders and hips (as viewed from the side). © 2009 Wolters Kluwer Health I Lippincott Williams and Wilkins.

My Neck Hurts!

head in a dish-shaped hollow. Lying on your side is also a good choice, but the pillow should be thicker to allow the neck to stay in a neutral position. Many products on the market can help you to maintain good posture during the day and in bed, such as seat supports, contoured pillows, and foot rests. Check with your physical therapist before purchasing any of these items to see what is best for your condition.

ULTRASOUND

Ultrasound is the transmission of sound waves through the mechanical vibration of a crystal within a sound head (device head; figure 3.44). The sound waves penetrate the skin by way of a coupling medium, either gel or water. Depending on the type of transmission, ultrasound can heat tissue or mechanically vibrate tissue. Ultrasound therapy is most effective when used to heat and relax the muscles and connective tissue prior to stretching.

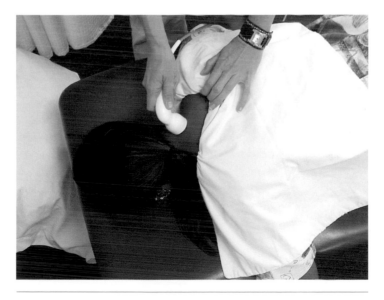

FIGURE 3.44 Demonstration of the use of ultrasound over the trapezius muscle.

How Physical Therapy Can Help

HEAT PACKS

Heat is a very effective and easily administered treatment for neck pain. It can reduce pain, muscle spasm, and inflammation, and it is especially helpful when used prior to stretching or traction. Moist heating pads or microwavable packs are recommended and should be applied prior to stretching (figure 3.45). At home, apply heat for no longer than 20 minutes and no more frequently than every 2 hours for up to 6 applications a day. Prolonged heat is not recommended because

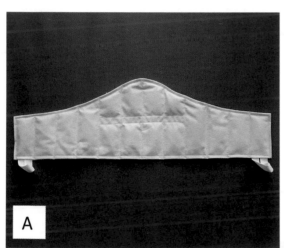

it can reverse the effects of the anti-inflammatory process. Take care when using an electric heating pad. These pads typically produce dry heat, which can more easily burn the skin.

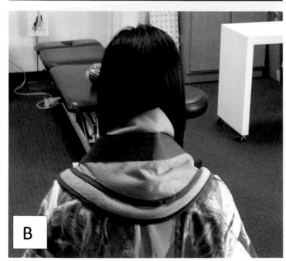

FIGURE 3.45   (A) Heat packs used in physical therapy are often made of clay encased in a thick cotton sleeve. They are stored in a hot water bath for moist heat. (B) Hot packs are wrapped in cloth for comfort and to prevent excessive heat or burning of the skin.

My Neck Hurts!

COLD PACKS AND ICE PACKS

Ice is not usually the preferred treatment for chronic neck pain, but it can be effective for acute, new-onset neck pain or strain. It is not recommended for tight or spastic muscles. Although commercial cold packs are available, ice from your freezer, placed in a plastic bag, is simple and effective. Avoid applying ice directly to the skin, which can be unpleasant. Place a thin towel or pillowcase, either slightly damp or dry, between your skin and the ice pack. Limit ice pack treatments to between 10 and 15 minutes maximum.

An ice massage can numb tender trigger points and can be administered with an ice cube or frozen water in a paper cup. The duration of treatment for ice massage is 5 to 8 minutes per area or until the areas are numb. The stages of sensation experienced prior to the numbness include cold, burning, and aching. The numbness is often a welcome relief from the pain.

IONTOPHORESIS AND PHONOPHORESIS

Iontophoresis is a modality used less often than some others. In iontophoresis, a medication, usually a steroid, is delivered into the muscle and connective tissue by means of an electrical current. A medicated cream is applied to the skin and absorption into the tissue is aided by mild electrical stimulation from an electrical pad. The goal of treatment is to reduce inflammation and to alleviate pain.

Phonophoresis is the delivery of a medication, usually hydrocortisone cream, into the muscle and connective tissue by means of an ultrasound transducer. This treatment method has the benefit of heating the tissue and aiding in absorption of medication at the same time.

ELECTRICAL STIMULATION

Treatments including transcutaneous electrical nerve stimulation (TENS) and sequential stimulation can be used as part of a therapy session. See chapter 4 for details on this modality.

CERVICAL TRACTION

Traction refers to the use of mechanical devices to relieve pressure on the skeletal system. Cervical traction can be a very effective method of treating chronic neck pain. It is designed to stretch the musculature of the neck as well as the cervical vertebral column to alleviate joint pressure, disc protrusion, or nerve impingement.

Two types of cervical traction devices are available for home use. The over-the-door models use a water bag (which can be filled to various weights) connected to a pulley system. With the person sitting in a chair, the water acts as a counter-balance to pull the neck up. Caution should be taken with this type of unit to avoid force under the chin or the jaw.

Pneumatic units, which allow the person to lie down, are more comfortable for those with chronic neck pain because the cervical musculature is more relaxed (figure 3.46). Conditions such as cervicogenic headaches, facet joint pain, cervical spondylolysis, osteoarthritis, cervical degenerative disc disease, and myofascial pain can all benefit from traction. Patients with rheumatoid arthritis may not be appropriate candidates for cervical traction because of a possible inflammatory instability of the spine.

Using a pneumatic unit, traction can be intermittent, by alternating 1 to 3 minutes of pressure with relaxation (pressure release) for 30 to 60 seconds, or static, with constant pressure for up to 5 to 10 minutes at a time. The traction should be increased to 25 pounds of force for best effect and should be administered at least once a day or, in some cases, even twice a day. I recommend intermittent traction using the

ComforTrac or Saunders pneumatic device, both of which have a pressure gauge that can be manually controlled (figure 3.47). This type of home traction device simulates the computerized model used in physical therapy programs. It also comes in its own carrying case for portability. With a physician's prescription, most people can have their insurance companies pay a portion or the entire cost of the unit.

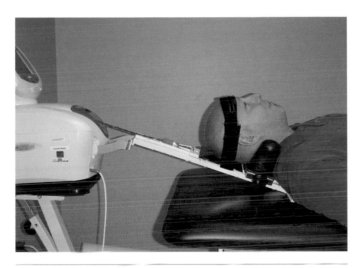

FIGURE 3.46   Home pneumatic units are most similar to this type of device, a computerized mechanical traction device used in a physical therapist's office.

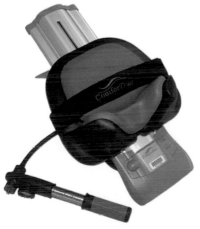

FIGURE 3.47   A home pneumatic traction device. Image courtesy of RS Medical. Used by permission.

How Physical Therapy Can Help

■ Back in Action with Traction

While directing traffic as part of his job as a deputy sheriff, Chris was struck by a car. The incident caused significant neck trauma, but he put off surgery for nearly eight years. He then underwent cervical fusion surgery, which had been recommended as the best way to address the neck and arm pain being caused by a herniated disc. But despite the surgery, his symptoms continued. "My neck pain and arm symptoms were no better after that." He retired, on full disability, soon after the surgery.

Years later, Chris learned that the vertebrae had never fused after the surgery, so a second surgery was planned. The "surgical revision" was performed, and after this intervention (plus physical therapy), he finally experienced relief from his symptoms and was able to stop using the narcotics his doctor had prescribed for pain.

Over time, Chris developed further degenerative disc disease at the level above his fusion, and eventually that disease began causing numbness and tingling in the arms, with worsening neck pain and grinding when he moved his neck. "The pain got worse, and after a while it was constant. It was severe with sharp stabbing jabs. When I'd turn my head, there was a grinding sound like two pine cones being rubbed together."

He saw his surgeon again, but it was decided to hold off on any more surgery in favor of conservative treatment. Chris was then referred to a physical medicine and rehabilitation doctor for further help.

The initial treatment prescribed was physical therapy. Chris had very limited range of motion in his neck, and his shoulders were weak. Treatments included heat application, intermittent cervical traction, gentle stretching, and range of motion exercises. After several weeks of therapy, his symptoms lessened significantly, and he had improved strength and the ability to perform daily activities. "Physical therapy helped the grinding and pain significantly. It reinforced the need for proper posture and daily exercises, and it allowed me to increase my daily activity as long as I continue doing what I was taught."

By the end of his physical therapy, he was able to purchase a pneumatic traction device to continue treatment at home, which helped maintain the gains he had made in weekly therapy sessions. Chris uses the traction device at home every day. Traction, along with stretching exercises and the occasional use of the pain relievers Relafen and Zanaflex, has dramatically changed his quality of life. The long-sought relief he gets from the regimen keeps him sticking to it. "People tell me that I don't look disabled. It's because I am religious about my daily stretches and proper posture. Plus, to avoid trouble, I limit my activity."

MANUAL THERAPY

Manual therapy is an important treatment but not all therapists offer it. A physical therapist with expertise in manual therapy has special skills that may enhance your range of motion and decrease your pain. Many of the techniques are borrowed from osteopathic and massage techniques. Chapter 5 provides detailed information about manual therapy and how these important techniques can help.

PHYSICAL THERAPY can at times seem tedious and can even temporarily increase your pain. But if you stay with it, you will find over time that it can alleviate pain and improve your ability to function in your daily activities. When exercise becomes part of your routine, you will gain strength and mobility, improved posture, and you may even develop a more optimistic outlook on life.

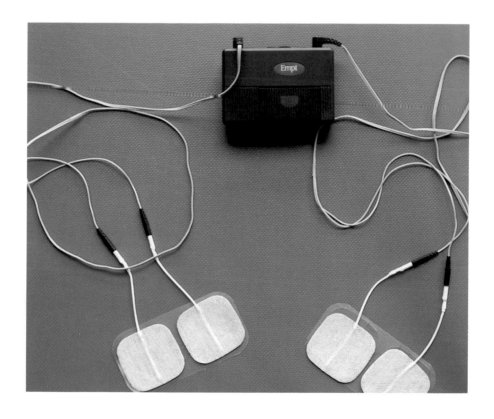

4

Electrical Treatments
Some Stimulating Options

You learned, no doubt at a young age, to avoid electrical shock, so it may be surprising to hear that electrical stimulation therapy is an important tool in treating chronic neck and upper back pain. These treatments range from noninvasive to permanent implants. Some are performed by physicians in an office, and some can be performed by the patient at home or even at work.

TRANSCUTANEOUS ELECTRICAL NERVE STIMULATION

One of the most commonly used electrical therapies is called TENS, which stands for transcutaneous (over the skin) electrical nerve stimulation. An electric pulse generator sends electrical impulses to electrode pads that have been adhered to the skin in the neck and upper back regions. This is considered a noninvasive treatment because there is no penetration of the skin. The pulse generator is approximately the size of a large cell phone and hooks easily onto a belt or waistband so that it can be used during daily activities. The unit has two channels with four self-adhesive, reusable pads that are made of silicone rubber.

The pads are placed directly over the painful muscles (figure 4.1). An electric field is produced over the skin without damaging it. After an initial application or instruction by your physician or physical therapist, you can use this treatment on your own. You control the level of electrical stimulation as well as the frequency and duration of the impulses (the device should not be turned up to the point where it is painful) It works by activating nerve fibers without producing muscle contraction. The unit is activated for at least one 30-minute session every 2 hours for a maximum of 8 hours per day. Pain relief can occur during stimulation and lasts for minutes to hours afterward.

TENS can provide long-term pain relief when used regularly. For

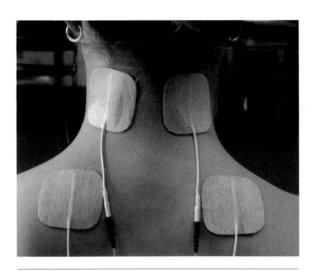

FIGURE 4.1   Typical placement of TENS unit pads on the neck and upper back.

My Neck Hurts!

most people, this portable device can improve their ability to perform daily activities with less discomfort. It can also be used for temporary symptom relief as part of a physical therapy session.

SEQUENTIAL STIMULATOR

Like a TENS unit, sequential stimulation units use an electric pulse generator to send electrical impulses to electrode pads placed on the surface of the skin over painful muscles. Sequential stimulator units differ from TENS by using an interferential stimulation that penetrates deeper into the tissue because it uses a higher frequency—4,000 to 5,000 Hz compared to 20 to 200 Hz for TENS. (Hz = hertz. One hertz is one cycle per second.) After 10 to 15 minutes of interferential treatment, a second phase of stimulation occurs, called muscle stimulation, which occurs at 71 Hz. Four channels (a total of eight pads) cover and stimulate a larger surface area and thus stimulate a larger area of tissue than TENS can. Sequential stimulation treatments can also provide longer pain relief than TENS after the stimulation is stopped.

The sequential stimulator unit is larger than a TENS unit. Although the unit is still small enough to be portable, treatments are typically administered at home. Each treatment lasts for an average of 30 to 45 minutes and can be used up to two times per day. Treatments are normally administered in a lying or seated position while watching television or reading. The pads can be adhered individually to the skin or incorporated into a vest. Vests are recommended for people with limited mobility or people who live alone, because a second person is usually needed to place the individual pads (figure 4.2).

PERCUTANEOUS NEUROMODULATION THERAPY

Percutaneous neuromodulation therapy (PNT) is minimally invasive electrical stimulation therapy. It was approved by the **Food and Drug**

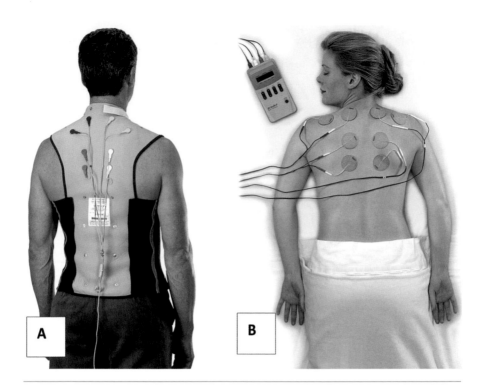

FIGURE 4.2   (A) Sequential stimulator vest. (B) Sequential stimulator for home use, demonstrated with eight pads over the entire upper back. Image courtesy of RS Medical. Used by permission.

Administration (FDA) in 2001 for use in the treatment of lower back pain and in 2002 for use in patients with chronic or intractable neck and upper back pain. PNT is often used after neck surgery or trauma in those who continue to experience chronic pain when more conservative treatments, such as physical therapy and medications, have failed. Studies of PNT have shown reduced pain, less use of pain medication, and improved ability to perform daily functions. The benefits of this therapy can continue for up to six months after the last treatment. Because this is a new therapy, it is unclear exactly how long users will experience continued improvement in symptoms. People with multiple diagnoses (including degenerative disc and joint disease, spinal steno-

My Neck Hurts!

sis, cervical strain, and fibromyalgia) and those with localized pain have responded to PNT in clinical trials.

The PNT system delivers electrical stimulation through fine-gauge filament electrodes (very small needles) that project from plastic safety casings called Safeguides. The Safeguides are placed on the skin, and the electrodes are inserted to a depth of 2 centimeters (approximately three-quarters of an inch) into the neck, shoulder, and upper back region (figure 4.3). The needles are so fine that they cause only minimal, brief discomfort when penetrating the skin; some people may feel

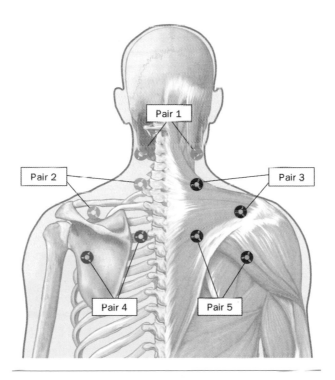

FIGURE 4.3 Standard placement of Safeguide electrodes in the neck and upper back region for percutaneous neuro-modulation therapy. Image courtesy of RS Medical. Used by permission.

mild discomfort at the site of the electrode insertion, but most do not. As a matter of fact, patients rarely report feeling the needles after they have been inserted.

Wires are connected to each Safeguide, and electrical stimulation is delivered into the muscle tissue. Nerves originating from the spinal cord pick up the electrical stimulation, which then affects the pain signals going to and coming from the brain (figure 4.4). Researchers believe that PNT stimulation calms the pain signals of the spinal cord nerve cells, which have become supersensitive in people with chronic pain. Studies have shown PNT to be effective for many individuals in reducing pain, improving activity levels, decreasing reliance on pain medications, and enhancing sleep. For most patients, the therapy is well tolerated, with little to no discomfort and few side effects.

Treatments are performed in a physician's office and last 30 to 45 minutes. The first several treatments are given weekly, at 5- to 10-day intervals; subsequent treatments are given less frequently because patients report longer periods of pain relief after multiple treatments.

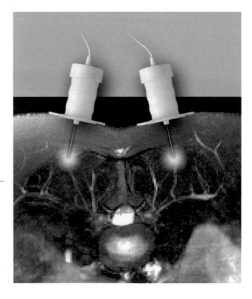

FIGURE 4.4   Cross-section view of the back, showing placement of PNT Safeguides with electrodes stimulating nerves in the back that travel to the spinal cord. Image courtesy of RS Medical. Used by permission.

My Neck Hurts!

Complications are rare. Bleeding or infection can occur, but both are rare. An allergic skin reaction to the glue on the Safeguides is also possible. In extremely thin individuals, a pneumothorax (punctured lung) is the most serious potential complication, but this is highly unlikely to occur given the small caliber and short length of the electrodes (2 centimeters). Safety of use during pregnancy has not been established. People with cardiac defibrillators are not eligible for PNT.

■ A PNT Success Story

Deborah is a 37-year-old account specialist for a local cable company. Her neck pain and headaches started after a car accident sixteen years ago. She experienced whiplash and mild head trauma when another car crashed into the passenger door of her car. The pain gradually disappeared over the course of a year, but about five years later, without any new accident or injury, she began experiencing neck and shoulder pain.

"It felt like someone was standing on my neck and shoulders, similar to when we formed a human pyramid as high school cheerleaders." Her symptoms were at first intermittent, but within several months, she developed daily pain, prompting her to see her primary care doctor. A muscle relaxant was prescribed, and she was encouraged to take over-the-counter pain relievers. She was also referred to a neurologist.

The neurologist gave her another type of muscle relaxant and treated her headaches with medication. Physical therapy was considered, but the frequent office visits did not fit into her schedule. She was referred to another neurologist for possible injection therapy.

She told the second neurologist, "The pain is almost intolerable. It's affecting every part of my life, work, and sleep." He ordered a medical workup that included a normal MRI of the head and cervical neck x-rays, which showed a reduced curve. Two rounds of trigger point injections were performed in the semispinalis cervicis, trapezius, rhomboid, and upper thoracic muscles. Each round of injections brought some pain relief, but for only two to three weeks at a time. Botulinum toxin therapy was then considered for longer relief from what was believed to be myofascial pain but her insurance company denied coverage for it.

Deborah wanted to avoid medications, and physical therapy still did not fit into her schedule. The neurologist recommended PNT. Treatments were given weekly for four weeks, and Deborah was pleased to find she experienced longer and longer pain relief with each session. Over time, her treatments were reduced to every eight weeks and are now being continued as maintenance. Her muscles get achy a few days before her next treatment is due. At her last visit, she told her neurologist, "I'm now taking much less medication for my neck pain, and even my headaches are better. I'm back to more of a normal life."

SPINAL CORD STIMULATION

Spinal cord stimulation (SCS) is a pain-control intervention in which electrical stimulation is applied directly over the spinal cord. Using implanted electrodes (see figure 4.5), an electric field is produced over the spinal cord that blocks pain impulses from being transmitted to the brain. This therapeutic option is considered a more invasive procedure and is an option only after surgery and all other major treatments have failed to adequately control pain.

Spinal cord stimulation (also known as dorsal column stimulation) was first approved by the FDA in 1989 as a therapy to address chronic pain. This treatment is thought to be most helpful for **neuropathic pain** (pain caused by damage or dysfunction of the nerves rather than by damage to the tissue). The goal of treatment is to reduce the patient's pain by 50 to 75 percent, while reducing or eliminating pain medications.

Although SCS is more commonly used in patients with low back or leg symptoms, lower neck and upper back and arm pain can also be treated successfully with this technique. It has been documented to aid in the management of chronic, intractable pain of the trunk and limbs, including unilateral or bilateral pain associated with the following conditions:

- arachnoiditis or lumbar adhesive arachnoiditis
- complex regional pain syndrome (reflex sympathetic dystrophy) or causalgia
- degenerative disc disease; herniated disc pain that has not been successfully addressed with conservative or surgical interventions
- epidural fibrosis
- failed back surgery syndrome (FBSS) or low back syndrome
- multiple back operations
- painful neuropathies
- post-laminectomy pain
- radicular pain syndrome or radiculopathies resulting from FBSS or herniated disc
- unsuccessful disc surgery

The placement of the electrodes along the spinal cord is determined by the site of symptoms. The electrodes are inserted through a small incision and then advanced under the skin to a place overlying the spinal cord membrane (dura mater). For neck, upper back, or arm pain, the electrodes are positioned in the cervical or upper thoracic region.

Stimulation of the spinal cord causes a tingling sensation in the region where pain was previously felt. While this tingling sensation may take some time to get used to, most people say it is better than the pain previously experienced.

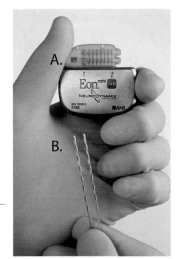

FIGURE 4.5   (A) A spinal cord stimulation generator and (B) electrodes. Image copyright St. Jude Medical, all rights reserved.

Electrical Treatments

To determine if you are a candidate for SCS, an initial stimulation test is performed with a temporary electrode and external pulse generator. An *on the table trial* entails the use of local anesthetic for electrode placement so that you can report the location of stimulation and if significant pain control is achieved. If the response is favorable, the permanent device is implanted by the doctor at that time.

Another alternative is called an *outpatient trial*, during which temporary electrodes are connected to an external pulse generator (about the size of a cell phone) worn outside the body while you go about your normal daily activities for several days. This is a more real-world test and can ensure efficacy before permanent implantation is considered.

The permanent implantable pulse generator sends the power signal though a wire (lead) to the electrode placed over the spinal cord. The pulse generator is placed under skin (in the abdomen or buttock) in a similar fashion to a pacemaker and can be programmed to maximum benefit using a handheld computer. The generator's battery typically lasts two to five years (depending on the pulse strength) before needing replacement.

The advantages of SCS include continuous pain relief without the potential side effects of other treatments such as medications. Since a minor surgical procedure is involved, there are risks, including bleeding, infection, spinal cord or nerve damage, and reaction to anesthetics. Once electrodes are in place, migration or movement can occur, resulting in loss of effectiveness. Patients with pacemakers or defibrillators are not candidates for spinal cord stimulation because of possible electrical interference between the devices. Having an MRI scan on any part of the body is not recommended in a patient with a spinal cord stimulator. The generator and electrodes as well as their implantation are also very expensive, and insurance companies may require that extensive criteria be met before they approve coverage.

ELECTRICAL STIMULATION is not an exclusive treatment for chronic pain. It is a therapy shown to be particularly effective for certain patients when used in conjunction with other treatments. Since its implementation ranges from noninvasive to the surgical implantation of a permanent device, it is usually best to begin with the simplest application and progress, if necessary, from there.

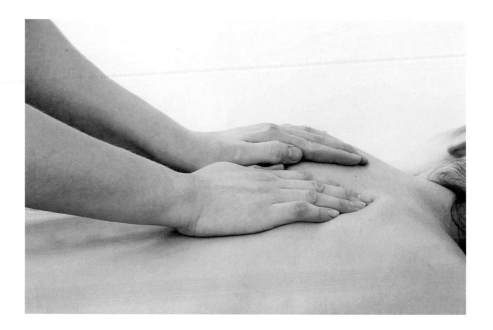

Manual Therapy

Hands-On Relief

M anual therapy is just what it sounds like—the use of hands-on treatment to relieve pain and encourage improved mobility and circula tion. This chapter provides an overview of the three most commonly accepted and prescribed forms of manual therapy. As a physician, I have recommended each of these therapies to patients over the years with significant success.

MASSAGE

Therapeutic massage involves the manual manipulation of the muscles, the **fascia** (the thin sheet of fibrous tissue that lies between the skin and muscles), and the skin over almost the entire body. For patients with chronic neck pain, massage is most helpful when applied to the muscles of the neck and upper back—the cervical, trapezius, levator scapulae, and rhomboid muscles. It can be especially useful in reducing localized muscular knots and trigger points.

Therapeutic massage is usually performed in a dimly lit room with soft music playing, creating an atmosphere that is intended to help reduce physical and emotional tension. If you have not yet had a professional massage, you should know that you are required to undress only to your comfort level; your sense of modesty is always respected. You will then lie down on the massage table under a sheet. Before touching your skin, the massage therapist applies a massage oil or lotion to his or her hands and then begins the treatment. A session lasts 30 to 90 minutes. Treatments can be given as frequently as two to three times per week for those with severe pain or as infrequently as once a month for maintenance or to address flare-ups or worsening pain.

Clinical research has demonstrated that therapeutic massage has benefits beyond the immediate local effects in the tissues treated. Evidence indicates that heart rate and blood pressure are reduced, the body's immune responses are boosted, and there is an increase in blood and lymphatic flow. A temporary sense of well-being and reduction of emotional stress is commonly reported. Like other manual therapies, massage has also been shown to reduce physical and physiological tension and increase the body's production of endorphins. Research studies have not been performed to evaluate massage specifically in the treatment of neck pain, but massage has been shown to give long-term benefits in other pain syndromes such as chronic low back pain, cancer-related pain, and headaches.

There are many types of massage, and different types incorporate different manual techniques. The most common is Swedish massage, which is a relatively gentle technique (figure 5.1). Pressure point therapy (Shiatsu) is a more direct treatment that focuses on relieving the pain and tension of trigger points (figure 5.2). It is similar to acupressure and myofascial release, which are performed by osteopaths

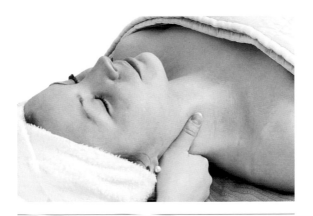

FIGURE 5.1   Traditional Swedish massage treating the cervical spinal muscles. © 2006 Tyler Olson. Image from BigStockPhoto.com.

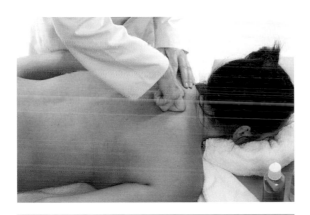

FIGURE 5.2   A massage therapist performing pressure point therapy in the region of the trapezius and levator scapulae muscles. © 2006 Leah-Anne Thompson. Image from BigStockPhoto.com.

and physical therapists. Sports massage focuses on muscle groups that can become tight and painful after exercise or from an activity that requires repetitive motions. Performed regularly, massage can be an important adjunctive therapy for chronic neck pain.

■ Rubbing Out the Pain

After carrying a mailbag for the U.S. Postal Service for seven years, Jon, then in his mid-forties, switched to a less physically demanding job in the mailroom, where he continues to work. For a few years he experienced a mild discomfort in his neck by the end of the day, and he took over-the-counter pain relievers such as Tylenol or Motrin in the evening.

About a year ago, the pain began starting earlier in the day, and it continued while he was at work. The symptoms were more pronounced on his left side, which was the shoulder he had carried his mailbag on for all those years. He made an appointment to see his primary care doctor, telling him, "I feel pretty good first thing in the morning, but as the work day progresses I get achy and tight."

An x-ray of the neck revealed no significant abnormalities, and he was given a prescription for Flexeril to reduce muscle spasm and pain. He was also advised to begin taking Celebrex (a nonsteroidal anti-inflammatory drug) daily as an alternative to Motrin because of his history of an ulcer and acid reflux. These medications helped somewhat, but Flexeril made him sleepy, so he took it only after getting home from work.

A co-worker suggested he see a massage therapist who had helped her with back pain. At first, he was reluctant to try this, thinking it was something only done at a spa. Eventually, he decided to give it a try and was pleasantly surprised. On his initial evaluation, the massage therapist noted tight muscles with multiple trigger points, especially on the left side, involving trapezius muscles, levator scapulae, and the rhomboids. During Jon's first session, the therapist performed deep tissue and trigger point massage, which relieved his pain and muscle spasms for a couple of days.

The therapist encouraged Jon to schedule regular weekly sessions to get the optimal benefit. After six weeks of treatment, Jon's symptoms were virtually gone. Now, he sees the therapist only as needed when there are flare-ups of the pain and tightness, which has been every other month or so.

"It's great to feel good all day long."

My Neck Hurts!

Certified massage therapists are regulated by state medical boards, and most therapists have received over 400 hours of classroom and practical training. Certification and practice standards are not present in all states, however. The American Massage Therapy Association is the largest association, with established practice standards and a code of professional ethics. No prescription is needed to see a massage therapist. Most massage therapy is not covered by insurance unless performed by a physical therapist, but in some states, a physician's prescription will allow for a discount or application of charges toward a flexible spending account. Visit www.amtamassage.org to learn more about massage and to find a certified massage therapist in your area.

OSTEOPATHIC MANIPULATIVE TREATMENT

Osteopathic physicians (D.O.s) and **allopathic physicians (M.D.s)** are the only fully licensed physicians in all fifty states to provide medical and surgical care. D.O.s represent all areas of medical specialties, from family practice to neurosurgery. Osteopathic training is more commonly focused on primary care, and therefore, more D.O.s practice in such areas as family practice, internal medicine, and pediatrics. The osteopathic philosophy promotes the body's own ability to heal itself, with the physician playing a supportive role in this process.

D.O.s receive 300 to 500 hours of additional training in a manual therapy called **osteopathic manipulative treatment (OMT)**, but not all D.O.s perform **manipulation** in their medical practice. Family medicine physicians make up the bulk of those performing OMT. A small number of D.O.s receive extra postgraduate training in manipulation and specialize in this therapy. Some allopathic physicians and physical therapists also receive training in OMT.

Osteopathic training in other countries covers only manipulative therapy, and therefore D.O.s from outside the United States do not practice as fully licensed physicians and are more like chiropractors in their scope of practice. This has led to public confusion and misunderstanding about what osteopathic physicians in the United States are trained to do. As noted, in the United States, D.O.s practice medicine like M.D.s do.

The practitioner can employ multiple osteopathic methods in treatment sessions to increase range of motion and to decrease pain and muscle spasm. Research studies regarding OMT are limited, but some studies show that patients receiving OMT recover faster than those using traditional medical therapy or physical therapy. This has been demonstrated in some patients with neck pain and fibromyalgia. In a study of patients with lower back pain, OMT resulted in a reduction in the amount of pain medicine used.

Side effects from OMT—which can include muscle stiffness and achiness, headaches, and dizziness—are rare. No serious complications have been reported except following high-velocity/low-amplitude (HVLA) manipulation of the neck. HVLA is the manipulative technique that most closely resembles chiropractic. (Chiropractic is discussed later in this chapter.) Unlike chiropractic, which centers on manipulation of the spinal column, osteopathic manipulation focuses on the myofascial tissue surrounding the spine. Most techniques involve gentle stretching and mobilization. Here is an overview of the most commonly performed techniques.

Counterstrain

In this technique, a tender muscular spot or trigger point is palpated firmly. At the same time, the head, neck, or arm is manually placed in the position causing the least amount of discomfort from the associated palpation. This position is held for about 90 seconds or until the tender point becomes less tender. The manipulated body part is then slowly placed back in its natural position.

Muscle Energy

The head, neck, or arm is manually positioned where muscular tension is felt. The patient then actively pushes against the practitioner for several seconds and then relaxes. When the physician feels a release in the patient's tissue, the tissue barrier is further manipulated to a new point of tension (figure 5.3). This is repeated several times to increase range of motion and decrease muscle spasm.

Myofascial (or Soft Tissue) Release

Myofascial release is a technique in which the hands of the practitioner are kept firmly on the skin (rather than sliding along the skin with the aid of an oil or cream, as in massage). The muscles and associated

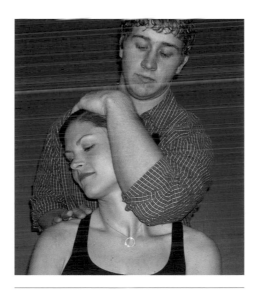

FIGURE 5.3 A demonstration of the muscle energy technique: The practitioner increases the lateral neck range of motion while the patient contracts and then relaxes her muscles against resistance.

fascia are stretched by the physician along the long axis and kneaded along the short axis of the muscle. The stretching action is guided by a release in muscular tension, which the practitioner feels as he or she applies pressure.

High-Velocity/Low-Amplitude

HVLA is the manipulative technique that most closely resembles chiropractic. It involves an extremely localized quick thrusting motion to mobilize a restricted joint but not typically beyond its normal range of motion.

CHIROPRACTIC

Chiropractic treatment is manipulation of the spine in an attempt to correct spinal misalignment, or to maintain correct alignment. **Chiropractors** use the term **subluxation** to describe the misalignment of the spine that can be felt by the practitioner but may not necessarily be seen on imaging studies such as x-ray or MRI. There is some controversy within the medical community regarding this concept because many allopathic physicians do not believe in subluxation as the cause of acute or chronic neck pain.

Chiropractors use a technique called an **adjustment** to treat pain or dysfunction of the neck or back (figure 5.4). The goal is to alleviate any irritation of spinal nerves and to improve spinal range of motion and alignment by correcting the subluxation. This maneuver consists of a high-velocity/low-amplitude thrust applied to a specific vertebral level. Localization to a certain cervical level is typically achieved by manually extending and rotating the neck followed by a quick thrust, mobilizing the specific vertebral joint past its normal anatomical range of motion. The thrust does not have to be particularly forceful for the treatment to be successful. A cracking or popping sound is often heard

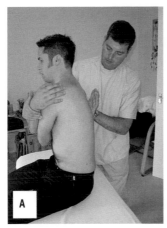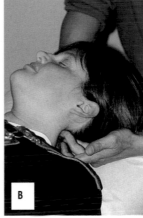

FIGURE 5.4   Positioning for chiropractic adjustments in the (A) upper back (thoracic) and (B) neck (cervical) areas. Image A: © 2006 Terence Walsh. Image B: © 2005 Fred Goldstein. Images from BigStockPhoto.com.

from a sudden release of oxygen, nitrogen, and carbon dioxide from facet joints, producing a vacuum. Elastic tissue and ligaments around the joint capsule are stretched, increasing range of motion.

For patients with neck pain, manipulation may also involve treatment of the low back or the pelvis to balance the entire spinal column. Balancing the pelvis may also include correcting any discrepancy in leg length difference by placing a heel lift in the shoe of the shorter leg. Initial treatments may be done as often as three to five times per week for the first two weeks, then tapering off based on the effectiveness of the therapy.

Treatments are well tolerated by most patients. Temporary complications of neck adjustments can include headaches, muscle achiness, and light-headedness or dizziness. More serious complications of cervical manipulation have been reported, but they are rare (1 per 400,000 to 3 per million treatments). They have included stroke, disc herniation, vertebral fracture or dislocation, quadriplegia, and even death. Because of these rare but possible risks, some physicians argue that cervical high-velocity manipulation should not be performed. Regardless, adjustments should *never* be performed on patients with a localized skin or bone infection or fracture, or in those with severe osteoporosis or severe arthritis (osteoarthritis or rheumatoid arthritis).

Chiropractors complete a bachelor's degree with an emphasis in science. Chiropractic training includes coursework in anatomy, physiology, pathology, nutrition, spinal manipulation, and chiropractic principles. Students graduating from such a program receive a doctor of chiropractic (D.C.) degree.

Chiropractors are regulated by the state in which they practice, and most states require proof of continuing medical education to maintain a license. Most private health insurance companies, Medicare, and workman's compensation cover chiropractic treatments, although Medicaid coverage varies by state.

Chiropractic treatment is considered by some to be an alternative or complementary form of medicine, but it is commonly sought at the first development of neck or back pain. Most of the research on chiropractic care has been on the treatment of low back pain. The results have been mixed, but there is some evidence of physiological and chemical effects from this type of manipulation. Increased blood flow and endorphin levels have been reported in some physiological studies. Clinical trials have demonstrated increased cervical range of motion, increased tolerance of pain, and reduction in muscle tension. No consistently reproducible vertebral disc retraction or stabilization has been demonstrated with manipulation.

Other therapies may be performed as part of a chiropractic treatment plan, including modalities offered by traditional physical therapists, such as heat application, ultrasound, traction, or decompression therapy, electrical stimulation, and exercise therapy. Many chiropractors also treat patients with dietary supplements or herbs and offer education on lifestyle changes to reduce pain. Some chiropractors are trained in **acupuncture**, a therapy that is described in chapter 8.

CERTIFIED MASSAGE THERAPISTS, osteopathic physicians, and chiropractors are dedicated health care professionals who have completed rigorous education and training before taking the state or national exams required for professional practice. It's important to find a credentialed practitioner with experience and expertise. Your doctor should be able to help you with a recommendation, but, if not, you will find help with that search in the last chapter of this book.

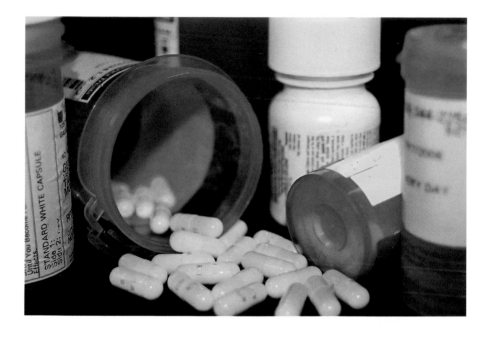

The Right Medications

M edications can be very helpful in reducing pain and muscles spasms in people with chronic neck and upper back pain. The right drug can improve the quality of your life not only by relieving your pain but also by treating other symptoms brought on by chronic pain such as sleeping problems, depression, and anxiety. While medication alone will not completely resolve most neck and upper back pain, when combined with other therapies, it plays an important role in achieving long-term improvement.

All drugs have potential side effects, but significant side effects tend to be more common with higher dosages. (The most common side effects for drugs frequently used to treat chronic pain are discussed in this chapter; mild side effects that occur may dissipate over time.) Your medications can be gradually increased to the maximum tolerated dose. This slow increase in medication dosage, called a **titration**, can take days to weeks, depending on the drug. For individuals with daily pain, this can be a frustrating process. Your doctor may have you try a number of medications until the best compound and dose are found to relieve your pain with minimal side effects.

NONSTEROIDAL ANTI-INFLAMMATORY DRUGS

Nonsteroidal anti-inflammatory drugs (NSAIDs) are the most commonly recommended medications for neck and upper back pain and are often the drug a physician will recommend first. This is partly due to the availability of over-the-counter medications such as aspirin, ibuprofen, and naproxen. These drugs have a dual action, reducing both pain and inflammation. The anti-inflammatory action can be maximized by regular dosing, which helps to maintain a consistent level of active ingredient in the patient's blood (called the *blood level*).

NSAIDs can be taken short term or long term and are usually well tolerated when used properly. Individuals with stomach or kidney problems need to be cautious when taking NSAIDs because of potential organ damage. People on blood thinners may also be poor candidates for NSAID therapy because these drugs can further reduce blood clotting to dangerous levels.

NSAIDs work by inhibiting cyclooxygenase-1 (COX-1) and cyclooxygenase-2 (COX-2). COX-1 inhibition leads to decreased blood platelet clumping, which can increase the risk of bleeding. This action can be beneficial for someone who has suffered from a heart attack or stroke, but it can lead to problems in others. COX-1 inhibition can also cause kidney problems in some people, especially if they have used NSAIDs excessively or for a long time.

A newer class of selective COX-2 inhibitors has recently come on the market. These drugs do *not* affect bleeding. They also have fewer gastrointestinal side effects and therefore may be a better choice for people with a history of ulcers or acid reflux disease. Unfortunately,

TABLE 6.1

FDA-approved dosages of nonsteroidal anti-inflammatory drugs (NSAIDs)

Generic name	Trade name	Pill strength (mg)	Dosage range (mg/day)
Aspirin	Bayer, Ecotrin	81, 325, 500	81–4,000
Celecoxib	Celebrex	100, 200, 400	200–800
Diclofenac potassium	Cataflam	25, 50	75–150
Diclofenac sodium	Voltaren Voltaren XR*	25, 50, 75 100 XR	75–225 100–200
Diflunisal	Dolobid	250, 500	500–1,000
Etodolac	Lodine	200, 300, 400, 500, 600 400 XL†, 500 XL, 600 XL	400–1,600
Flurbiprofen	Ansaid	50, 100	200–300
Ibuprofen	Advil, Motrin, Nuprin, Rufen	200, 400, 600, 800	600–3,600
Indomethacin	Indocin	25, 50, 75 SR‡	75–225
Ketoprofen	Orudis, Actron Oruvail	12.5, 25, 50, 75 200 SR	50–300 200
Ketorolac tromethamine	Toradol	10	10–40
Meclofenamate	Meclomen	50, 100	200–400
Mefenamic acid	Ponstel	250	500–1,000
Meloxicam	Mobic	7.5, 15	7.5–15
Nabumetone	Relafen	500, 750	1,000–2,000
Naproxen	Naprosyn, Aleve	250, 375, 500	500–1,500
Oxaprozin	Daypro	600	600–1,200
Piroxicam	Feldene	10, 20	20
Salsalate	Disalcid, Salflex	500, 750	3,000
Sodium naproxen	Anaprox	275, 550	550–1,100
Sulindac	Clinoril	150, 200	300–400
Tolmetin sodium	Tolectin	200, 400, 600	600–1,800

Note: For patients with more severe symptoms, physicians may prescribe higher daily dosages than those approved by the FDA.

*XR = extended release

†XL = extended release

‡SR = sustained release

concerns have arisen regarding this class of medications and a possible associated increased risk for cardiovascular disease. In fact, two popular COX-2 inhibitors, Vioxx and Bextra, have been taken off the market in the United States because of these concerns.

The FDA has expressed concerns that all NSAIDs may cause an increased risk of cardiovascular thrombotic events and stroke (with the exception of aspirin). It is not recommended that NSAIDs be combined. Aspirin should not be used in children due to the risk of Reye syndrome.

NARCOTIC ANALGESICS (OPIOIDS)

Narcotics, such as Vicodin and Percocet, can provide temporary pain relief and can be helpful in times of worsening pain. Combination pills that contain acetaminophen or ibuprofen to boost pain-relieving effectiveness are also available. Long-term use of narcotics for chronic neck and upper back pain is somewhat controversial because of the potential for addiction. In most cases, narcotics can be used for those times when pain worsens (physicians refer to this as *breakthrough pain*), or when other treatments are not as helpful as desired, usually in relation to increased physical activity. This "as needed" use of narcotics is preferable to a daily dosage for the majority of patients.

There are occasions, however, when daily use of narcotics can be appropriate, such as with compression fractures, severe arthritis, spine cancer, and continued pain after surgical intervention. For people with these pain syndromes, narcotics are dosed regularly to maintain a consistent blood level and can even be delivered by an implanted pump. A daily use of narcotics should be considered only when pain is debilitating and after other options have been exhausted. Patients must follow strict instructions, and some physicians even require a signed contract to ensure compliance. Intermittent blood tests may be ordered to determine drug levels, allowing the doctor to monitor the patient and avoid abuse.

TABLE 6.2
FDA-approved dosages of narcotic analgesics (opioids)

Generic name	Trade name	Pill strength (mg)	Dosage range (mg/day)
Codeine	None	15, 30, 60	90–3,600
Hydromorphone	Dilaudid	1, 2, 3, 4	6–12
		3 (suppositories)	6–12
Levorphanol	Levo-Dromoran	2	2–8
Meperidine	Demerol	50, 100	50–900
Methadone	Dolophine	5, 10	20–80
Morphine	MSIR	15, 30	30–180
Morphine CR*	MS Contin	15, 30, 60, 100, 200	30–200
Morphine SR⁺	Kadian	20, 30, 50, 60, 100	20–200
	Avinza	30, 60, 90, 120	30–120
Oxycodone	Roxicodone	5	10–20
	OxyContin (CR)	10, 20, 40	10–80
Oxymorphone	Opana	5, 10	5–120
	Opana ER‡	5, 7.5, 10, 15, 30, 40	5–120
Propoxyphene	Darvon	32, 65	65–390

Note: For patients with more severe symptoms, physicians may prescribe higher daily dosages than those approved by the FDA.
*CR = controlled release   †SR = sustained release   ‡ER = extended release

TABLE 6.3
FDA-approved dosages of narcotic analgesic combinations

Generic name	Trade name	Pill strength (mg/mg)	Pills per day
Codeine and acetaminophen	Tylenol with Codeine	15/300, 30/300, 60/300	1–2 every 4 hours
Codeine and aspirin	Empirin with Codeine	30/325, 60/325	1–2 every 4 hours
Hydrocodone and acetaminophen	Anexsia, Lorcet Lortab	5/500, 7.5/650 2.5/500, 5/500, 7.5/500, 10/500	1–2 every 4–6 hours 1–2 every 4–6 hours
	Vicodin	5/500	1–2 every 4–6 hours
	Vicodin ES*	7.5/750	1 every 4–6 hours
Oxycodone and acetaminophen	Percocet	5/325	1 every 6 hours
	Tylox	5/500	1 every 6 hours
Oxycodone and aspirin	Percodan	5/325	1 every 6 hours
Propoxyphene and acetaminophen	Darvocet N-50	50/325	1–2 every 4–6 hours
	Darvocet N-100	100/650	1 every 4–6 hours
	Wygesic	65/650	1 every 4 hours

Note: For patients with more severe symptoms, physicians may prescribe higher daily dosages than those approved by the FDA. Total acetaminophen dose should not exceed 4,000 mg per day.
*ES = extra strength

Why all the concern? Long-term use of narcotics for chronic pain can lead to physical dependence (addiction), and the user's tolerance will change too, requiring higher and higher doses over time to achieve the desired effect. Common side effects include sedation and constipation. Fortunately, there are other types of medication that may, when combined with other treatments, provide better and safer long-term relief from pain.

ANTISEIZURE MEDICATIONS

Antiseizure medications (**anticonvulsants**) reduce pain by diminishing nerve impulses and relaxing muscles. Some of these drugs can also improve sleep and decrease depression and anxiety. Associated pain and tingling sensations that radiate into the arms and that are

TABLE 6.4
FDA-approved dosages of antiseizure medications

Generic name	Trade name	Pill strength (mg)	Dosage range (mg/day)
Carbamazepine	Tegretol	100, 200	200–1,600
	Tegretol XR*	100, 200, 400	
	Carbatrol	100, 200, 300	
Gabapentin	Neurontin	100, 300, 400, 600, 800	300–3,600
Lacosamide	Vimpat	50, 100, 150, 200	100–400
Lamotrigine	Lamictal	25, 100, 150, 200	100–250
Levetiracetam	Keppra	250, 500, 750	500–3,000
Pregabalin	Lyrica	50, 75, 100, 150, 300	100–600
Oxcarbazepine	Trileptal	150, 300	600–2,400
Tiagabine	Gabitril	2, 4, 8, 12, 16, 24	4–56
Topiramate	Topamax	15, 25, 50, 100	25–400
Valproic Acid	Depakote	125, 250, 500	500–4,000
	Depakote ER†	250, 500	
Zonisamide	Zonegran	25, 50, 100	100–600

Note: For patients with more severe symptoms, physicians may prescribe higher daily dosages than those approved by the FDA.
*XR – extended release
†ER = extended release

My Neck Hurts!

related to neck pain can be reduced significantly with antiseizure medications.

Antiseizure medications are most helpful in treating nerve-related (neuropathic) pain, but other types of pain can also be helped with these drugs. Gabapentin (Neurontin) and pregabalin (Lyrica) may be the most commonly used medications in this class to treat pain. They are the only oral medications approved by the FDA to treat the neuropathic pain condition associated with shingles known as postherpetic neuralgia. Depakote and Topamax are approved by the FDA for the prevention of migraine headaches. Lyrica is also approved for management of fibromyalgia symptoms.

The prescription of any antiseizure medicine to treat neck pain is considered an **off-label** use. This means that the medication is FDA approved for another condition or other conditions but has not been approved for use in pain relief. In January 2008, the FDA placed an alert that antiseizure drugs increased the risk of suicidal behavior and suicidal thoughts.

ANTIDEPRESSANTS

Tricyclic antidepressant medications are the oldest class of antidepressants and are used to treat many painful conditions. They are believed to be better at treating pain than many of the newer classes of antidepressants, but they also typically have more side effects, which can include sleepiness, dry mouth, constipation, urinary retention, and weight gain. These medications are taken at night to reduce side effects and to aid in sleep. Newer antidepressants (such as Prozac and Paxil) can be helpful, but they do not seem to be as effective for the treatment of pain. Cymbalta and Savella have been approved for management of fibromyalgia symptoms. **Antidepressants** can chemically help to calm the nerves that cause pain as well as to improve mood.

In 2004, the FDA issued a public health warning of an increased risk of suicidal thoughts and actions associated with the use of anti-

TABLE 6.5
FDA-approved dosages of antidepressants

Generic name	Trade name	Pill strength (mg)	Dosage range (mg/day)
Tricyclic antidepressants			
Amitriptyline	Elavil	10, 25, 50, 75, 100, 150	10–300
Clomipramine	Anafranil	25, 50, 75	25–250
Desipramine	Norpramin	10, 25, 50, 75, 100	10–300
Doxepin	Sinequan	10, 25, 50, 75, 100, 150	10–300
Imipramine	Tofranil	10, 25, 50, 75, 100, 125, 150	10–300
Nortriptyline	Pamelor	10, 25, 50, 5	10–250
Selective serotonin reuptake inhibitors (SSRIs)			
Citalopram	Celexa	10, 20, 40	10–40
Escitalopram	Lexapro	5, 10, 20	10–20
Fluoxetine	Prozac	10, 20	20–40
Fluvoxamine	Luvox	50, 100	100–300
Paroxetine	Paxil	20, 30	20–50
Sertraline	Zoloft	25, 50, 100	50–200
Serotonin-norepinephrine reuptake inhibitors (SNRIs)			
Desvenlafaxine succinate	Pristiq	50, 100	50–400
Duloxetine	Cymbalta	20, 30, 60	30–60
Milnacipran hydrochloride	Savella	12.5, 25, 50, 100	100–200
Venlafaxine	Effexor	25, 37.5, 50, 75, 100	75–225
	Efferor XR*	37.5, 75, 150	75–225
Norepinephrine-dopamine reuptake inhibitors			
Bupropion	Wellbutrin	75, 100	75–450
	Wellbutrin SR[+]	100, 150, 200	100–450
	Wellbutrin XL[‡]	150, 300	150–450
Serotonin antagonists and reuptake inhibitors			
Nefazodone	Serzone	100, 150, 200, 250	100–600
Trazodone	Desyrel	50, 100, 150, 200	50–600

TABLE 6.5 (*continued*)

Generic name	Trade name	Pill strength (mg)	Dosage range (mg/day)
Norepinephrine and serotonin antagonists			
Mirtazapine	Remeron	15, 30	15–45

Note: For patients with more severe symptoms, physicians may prescribe higher daily dosages than those approved by the FDA.
*XR = extended release
†SR = sustained release
‡XL = extended release

depressants in children or young adults up to age 24 during initial treatment. No statement of concern has been made regarding the use of antidepressants in adults older than 24.

MUSCLE RELAXANTS

Muscle relaxants such as Flexeril, Zanaflex, and Klonopin can be very helpful in reducing pain associated with muscle spasms. These medications are usually started at low doses to avoid side effects, the most common of which are sleepiness or dizziness (see Table 6.6).

MISCELLANEOUS MEDICATIONS

Because of their unique mechanisms of action, some medications do not fall into one single category. One such drug is tramadol (Ultram), which has a weak opioid effect as well as an action to increase available serotonin and norepinephrine. The combination of tramadol and acetaminophen (Ultracet) has similar pain-relieving effects as codeine with acetaminophen, only with fewer side effects. Tramadol has little to no addictive potential compared with narcotics. The most common side effects are nausea, dizziness, sleepiness, and headache. It may also decrease the threshold of having a seizure in patients who

TABLE 6.6
FDA-approved dosages of muscle relaxants

Generic name	Trade name	Pill strength (mg)	Dosage range (mg/day)
Baclofen	Lioresal	10, 20	30–80
Carisoprodol	Soma	350	350–1,400
Chlorphenesin	Maolate	400	1,600–2,400
Chlorzoxazone	Parafon Forte Paraflex	250, 500	1,500–2,000
Clonazepam	Klonopin	0.5, 1, 2	1–20
Cyclobenzaprine hydrochloride	Flexeril	5, 10	15–60
Diazepam	Valium	2, 5, 10	5–40
Metaxalone	Skelaxin	400, 800	2,400–3,200
Methocarbamol	Robaxin	500, 750	1,500–6,000
Orphenadrine citrate	Norflex Norgesic	100	100–200
Tizanidine hydrochloride	Zanaflex tablets Zanaflex capsules	2, 4 2, 4, 6	2–36 2–36

Note: For patients with more severe symptoms, physicians may prescribe higher daily dosages than those approved by the FDA.

are prone to seizures. Ultram is supplied in 50 mg pills, with a recommended daily dose of 50 to 400 mg per day. Each Ultracet pill contains 37.5 mg of tramadol and 500 mg of acetaminophen, and one to two pills are recommended every 4 to 6 hours as needed. A long-acting formula of tramadol is available (Ultram ER, in 100 mg, 200 mg, and 300 mg pills); it needs to be taken only once per day.

Tapentadol (Nucynta) acts as both an opioid analgesic and a norepinephrine reuptake inhibitor. It comes in 50, 75, and 100 mg tablets used up to 600 mg per day. Nausea, dizziness, constipation, and sedation are the most commonly reported side effects.

Embeda is a novel drug compound that combines morphine, an opioid analgesic, with naltrexone, which is an "anti"-opioid. This drug was specifically designed to prevent narcotic abuse by those crushing a pill to achieve a high due to quicker absorption. The naltrexone is only active if the pill is crushed, negating the action of the morphine. Pill strengths include (morphine/naltrexone) 20 mg/0.8 mg, 30 mg/1.2 mg, 50 mg/2 mg, 60 mg/2.4 mg, 80 mg/3.2 mg, and 100 mg/4 mg.

Oral corticosteroids (such as prednisolone and methylprednisolone) can be used for a short time to break a cycle of pain thought to be caused by inflammation in the tissues. Short-term use usually means one to two weeks. Used in this way, these drugs can give temporary or more long-term relief depending on the severity of the condition. Corticosteroids are very safe when used for a short time. The most common side effects are insomnia, water retention, upset stomach, and a feeling of energy, agitation, or irritability. Long-term steroid use is not a viable option because of potentially more serious side effects when used for months to years. Corticosteroids are not the same as anabolic steroids, which are illegal and are typically used by body builders or athletes.

TOPICAL MEDICATIONS

Capsaicin cream (Capzasin-P, Dolorac, Zostrix) is an over the-counter preparation made from the seeds of the chili pepper. The medication is applied to the skin in the painful region several times per day. It may take up to two weeks of regular application to experience relief. Pain may actually increase temporarily until the cream takes effect. Capsaicin works by depleting sensory nerve cells of a chemical (substance P) that is involved in pain transmission to the spinal cord.

Fentanyl transdermal (Duragesic) is a narcotic patch that allows the drug to be absorbed continuously through the skin into the bloodstream. Side effects can be similar to those of oral narcotics, but sedation occurs less frequently. Nausea or vomiting can limit its use, but these side effects tend to be a problem only with higher doses. Other side effects can include constipation, sweating, dry mouth, restlessness, nervousness, confusion, weight loss, or dizziness. A new patch is placed on the skin every three days (72 hours), making it convenient to use. It can also be a good option for those who have a problem taking oral medication. Patch dosages include 25, 50, 75, and 100 micrograms per hour.

Lidocaine 5% patch (Lidoderm Patch) is a large patch (10 cm x 14 cm, or approximately 4 inches by 5.5 inches) containing an anesthetic, which can be placed on the skin over a painful region (figure 6.1). It was approved by the FDA for shingles pain, but clinicians have found it useful off-label in other painful conditions. The package insert recommends placing the patch over the painful area for up to 12 hours. Some physicians suggest keeping the patch on for up to 24 hours at a time for the best result. Side effects are very uncommon, and the patch can be used along with oral medications. It is possible to have an allergic reaction to the medication or the glue in the patch. Some people also have difficulty getting the patches to stick well to the skin.

Diclofenac epolamine 1.3% topical patch (Flector) looks similar to Lidoderm, but each patch contains 180 mg of the NSAID diclofenac. The medication is absorbed into the skin and muscle tissue. The patch is FDA approved for up to a total daily dose of 360 mg, which equals

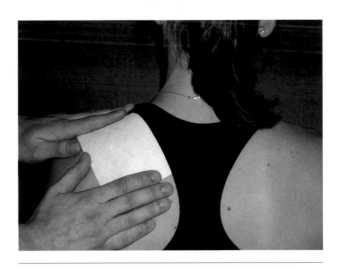

FIGURE 6.1 Lidoderm Patch placed over the upper back, across the shoulder blade.

My Neck Hurts!

one patch placed over a painful area every 12 hours. On-label use is for an acute sprain or injury. Physicians commonly prescribe more than one patch at a time for chronic pain. Similar side effects seen with oral NSAIDs are possible, but gastrointestinal upset is much less likely. Oral NSAIDs can be used along with the Flector patch.

Menthol with methyl salicylate (Ben-Gay, Icy Hot) or menthol alone (peppermint oil) is used in over-the-counter topical preparations including creams and patches. They can provide modest pain relief if applied regularly to the skin. Methyl salicylate is a topical form of a medication similar to aspirin. Another topical aspirin-like product is trolamine salicylate, which is found in over-the counter preparations such as Aspercreme and Myoflex.

IT IS ONLY NATURAL to commiserate with others who seem to be experiencing the same pain, but you should not assume that the medication a friend is using will help you or that it's even safe for you to try it Always consult with your physician first. And if in your travels you learn of a drug that seems to have good results, share the information with your doctor. You just may have some news on a promising medication before he or she does.

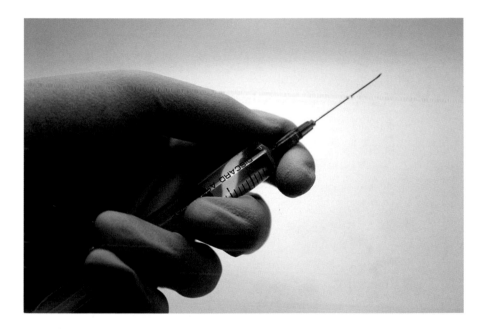

Getting to the Point with Injection Therapy

When more conservative treatments, such as physical therapy, manual therapy, or medication, have failed to provide satisfactory pain relief, or if you have an area of persistent spasm or tightness in the neck or shoulder muscles, there is another approach to consider—injection therapy. Although it is not as well known as the treatment options reviewed in earlier chapters, injection therapy is fairly routine and causes only temporary discomfort when performed by a skilled physician.

TRIGGER POINT INJECTIONS

Painful muscles may have associated trigger points. People with chronic muscle pain in the neck, shoulder, and

105

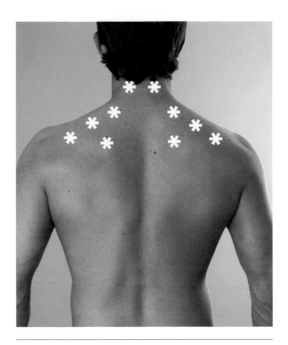

FIGURE 7.1   Common locations for trigger point injections in the neck and shoulder region. © 2007 Fred Goldstein. Image from BigStockPhoto.com.

upper back tend to have more than one trigger point. These painful areas, which can result from muscle strain, injury, or chronic inflammation, feel like a tight band, a tender spot, or a knot in the muscle. Injections of anesthetic or steroids into trigger points can temporarily help reduce muscle-related pain in medically appropriate candidates (figure 7.1).

The procedure usually takes only a few minutes. A fine needle is inserted into several areas of the painful muscle. A small amount of anesthetic or steroid (or both) is injected into each trigger point to relax the muscle and reduce pain. Most people report experiencing only minor, temporary discomfort. To reduce discomfort from the procedure, some physicians apply an anesthetic cold spray over the skin before injecting. If your anticipation of the pain is making you anxious, ask your doctor about this option.

After the injections are performed, the patient should take it easy for the rest of the day. The injected muscles may be sore for one to two days. The application of moist heat or ice can help reduce achiness if it occurs. Keep in mind that it can take up to 24 to 36 hours to notice a reduction in muscle pain. Clinical experience suggests that patients who respond well to trigger point injections experience a decrease in pain and muscle tightness and spasm for four weeks on average. Some people report even longer relief.

BOTULINUM TOXIN THERAPY

Botulinum toxin is a biological protein produced by the bacteria *Clostridium botulinum*. For medical procedures, the toxin is purified of all bacterial traces. When small amounts are injected into muscles, it can effectively reduce spasm and pain.

Injections of botulinum toxin are similar to trigger point injections but they tend to provide longer pain relief for patients with chronic neck and back pain. Botulinum toxin prevents the action of nerve chemicals crossing from nerve endings to muscle (figure 7.2). It also

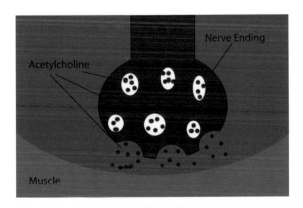

FIGURE 7.2 Diagram of a nerve-muscle junction. Botulinum toxin blocks the release of the neuro-chemical acetylcholine from the nerve terminal, which prevents muscle contraction.

blocks the release of nerve chemicals directly involved in the transmission of pain.

Botox (botulinum toxin type A) is the most common form of botulinum toxin used medically in the United States today. It was first approved by the FDA in 1989 for treatment of strabismus (crossed eyes or wall eyes), blepharospasm (uncontrolled eyelid blinking), and hemifacial spasm. It was approved for the treatment of cervical dystonia (torticollis) in 2000 and for facial wrinkles in 2002 (the discovery of its effectiveness in this regard was accidental). Cervical dystonia is an abnormal posturing of the head from twisting or turning of the neck, a condition also commonly associated with neck pain and tremor. In initial trials, Botox was used primarily to treat this type of head turning and head tremor. It quickly became apparent, however, that patients were also receiving significant pain relief with Botox injections. Currently, Botox is the treatment of choice for patients who suffer from cervical dystonia. Myobloc (botulinum toxin type B) is also available in the United States and was approved in 2002 for cervical dystonia only. A second type of botulinum toxin type A (Dysport) was approved by the FDA in 2009 for treating torticollis as well as facial wrinkles.

One of the most common uses of botulinum toxin is in patients experiencing the effects of a previous stroke, cerebral palsy, or multiple sclerosis. These conditions commonly cause a great deal of muscle spasm in the affected limb or limbs, which can cause flexion and pain. Botulinum toxin injections can reduce spasm-related pain, in addition to improving function. Injections can also be used to treat tremor, writer's cramp, and even motor tics. These uses along with treating pain are considered off-label. Research on the use of botulinum toxin to treat other painful conditions involving tight or spastic muscles that cause pain and other symptoms is ongoing. Some studies as well as personal clinical experience have demonstrated excellent effect in treating neck and upper back pain in the appropriate candidate.

Injection of the botulinum toxin takes only a few minutes. The injections are similar to those for trigger points, but they may be given deeper into the painful muscle. An electromyography (EMG) machine may be used to determine the best location for injection.

The needle used is small, but there is slight discomfort when it enters the muscle. Bruising or soreness can occur at the site. Some patients may develop a mild fever, malaise, and fatigue (resembling a flulike illness) for a few days following the injections, but this is very uncommon. A *temporary* excessive weakness can occur in the muscle at or around the injection site. Those patients who are injected in and around the neck sometimes experience heaviness in the head.

Botulinum toxin treatment takes effect in about two to five days after injection and usually lasts an average of three to three and a half months. Repeated injections tend to give better results. Many people are first treated with trigger point injections and later progress to botulinum toxin injections. A temporary response to trigger point injections may predict a longer and typically better response to Botox, Myobloc, or Dysport.

■ Back to Work with Botox
Donna, a 43-year-old executive assistant had been suffering from neck pain for fifteen years by the time she sought medical treatment. X-rays and MRI of her neck did not show any major abnormalities. Her pain had not started with a trauma or injury, and Donna believed that her work in a busy medical office, which required her to be at a desk all day—and with less than ideal ergonomics- was the cause of her pain or, at least, a contributor.

The pain brought on daily headaches and even migraines: "By the end of an eight-hour day, my neck was so painful and tight that it hurt just to turn and greet patients." Yet no one was able to find a reason or make a diagnosis. This caused Donna a lot of frustration, a factor that added to her cycle of pain. Some people even implied that perhaps it was "all in her head." Donna tried physical therapy, and it helped, but for numerous reasons she wasn't able to stay with it on an ongoing basis. She also tried chiropractic treatment, which she quickly abandoned because it made her symptoms worse.

Her family doctor eventually diagnosed myofascial pain and prescribed pain medications. But Donna didn't like the drowsiness and fatigue they caused. A subsequent referral to a neurologist led to trigger point injections using steroids. These treatments gave her some relief for up to several weeks at a time. She also adjusted the position of her computer at work, and that seemed to help things, too. Now, getting the first real relief she'd experienced in years, she was more determined than ever to free herself from chronic pain.

Some months later, she made an appointment with another neurologist for a second opinion. She laughed when the physician suggested botulinum toxin therapy with Botox. "I thought that was for facial wrinkles!" But she agreed to try it. "The Botox injections were a life-changing experience. I wished I had known about this years ago." Her neck and upper back pain relief was tremendous, with almost complete elimination of her headaches for up to three months.

Donna now receives injection treatments every three months, and she usually knows she's due for an injection one or two weeks in advance because muscle spasms and migraine headaches begin to crop up. Donna has not had any side effects from Botox injections and plans to continue the treatments. "I am so happy to finally be pain free. Being able to complete a full day of work without pain, or side effects from medications, has been amazing. I finally feel normal again."

Patients who are pregnant, trying to get pregnant, or breastfeeding are *not* eligible to receive botulinum toxin treatments. Other people who should *not* have botulinum toxin treatment include those with myasthenia gravis or Eaton-Lambert syndrome, or patients taking aminoglycoside antibiotics.

On April 30, 2009, the FDA issued a "black box" warning for all botulinum toxins, noting that the action was necessary due to reports that "the effects of botulinum toxin may spread from the area of injection to other areas of the body, causing symptoms similar to those of botulism, including unexpected loss of strength or muscle weakness, hoarseness or trouble talking, trouble saying words clearly, loss of bladder control, trouble breathing, trouble swallowing, double vision,

My Neck Hurts!

blurred vision, and drooping eyelids. These symptoms have been reported in children with cerebral palsy being treated with the products for muscle spasticity and in cases of unapproved use of the drugs. Symptoms have also been reported in adults treated both for approved and unapproved uses."

OCCIPITAL NERVE BLOCKS

Occipital nerve blocks are performed to reduce pain and abnormal sensations (tingling, pins and needles) from irritation of or damage to an occipital nerve (occipital neuralgia). This condition is common in patients with chronic neck pain and causes symptoms at the base of the skull that radiate into the top and sides of the head (see chapter 2).

Occipital nerve blocks are similar to trigger point injections. Anesthetics or steroids (or both) are injected around the area of one or both occipital nerves (figure 7.3). A small needle is typically used for an

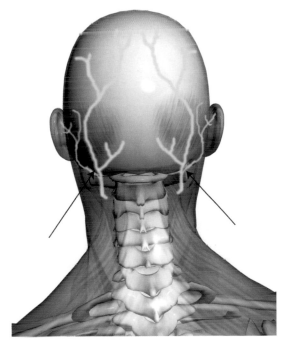

FIGURE 7.3   Typical location of an occipital nerve block. © 2005 Patrick Hermans. Image from BigStockPhoto.com.

injection made at the base of the skull after the area is cleaned with alcohol or iodine. The patient is usually in a seated position, and the procedure takes only a few minutes. Medication injected between the skull and scalp bathes the branches of the occipital nerves. The back and side of the head on the injection side will become numb for up to several hours depending on the type of anesthetic used. This sensation does not cause sleepiness or difficulty thinking. A small amount of soreness or swelling can occur after the injection, which can be treated with an ice pack if needed. The injections can help reduce pain in the back of the head and even upper neck for several weeks.

■ Sideswiped but not Sidelined

Clarice was a 29-year-old medical assistant who had enjoyed good health and had never had a medical problem—until the car she was riding in was sideswiped on the driver's side. The impact pushed the driver all the way over to the passenger side of the car, knocking heads with Clarice.

Initially, she didn't seek medical treatment. Later that night, though, she began to experience pain and muscle spasms in her neck and shoulders, which continued the next day. She also developed intermittent pain that radiated from her neck into her head.

Although Clarice hoped the pain would disappear over the next few days, it did not. So, two weeks after the accident, she met with a chiropractor. X-rays revealed some loss of curve in the cervical spine, and a diagnosis of sprain and strain was made. The chiropractor performed spinal manipulation complemented with electrical stimulation and hot packs three times a week for about a month. After that, the frequency of treatment was decreased, and by the second month, Clarice had achieved significant relief, particularly in the improved range of motion in her neck. "It was great to finally get movement back in my neck, but manipulation didn't do much for my pain."

Because of the ongoing pain, Clarice was referred to a physical medicine and rehabilitation physician (physiatrist), who prescribed a week of oral steroids to reduce inflammation and to break the cycle of pain. This treatment did give relief, but only for about two weeks.

My Neck Hurts!

By the fourth month after the accident, Clarice's range of motion and overall condition were much better, but she remained frustrated by the continuing neck pain and headaches. She was opposed to the suggestion of taking daily pain relievers because of her concerns about potential side effects. "Pain relief was very important to me, but I had to function. And I didn't want to miss work due to my pain or the effects of medication." It was at this point that Clarice was referred to a neurologist.

After a thorough evaluation, the neurologist determined that Clarice was a good candidate for injection therapy. A combination of trigger point injections and occipital nerve block almost completely resolved her pain for about six weeks. After a second round of injections, she found that she had only "occasional achiness or pain" in her neck and rarely had headaches. When she does experience a flare-up of pain or a spasm, she uses a TENS (transcutaneous electrical nerve stimulation) unit at home to address it. "Injections really reduced my neck pain and headaches. Plus, it's great being able to go to work and live my daily life without feeling the side effects from pain medication."

FACET BLOCKS (MEDIAL BRANCH BLOCKS)

Facet joint arthritis or trauma to the facet joint can cause significant neck pain that radiates down the shoulders and arms and that may not respond to more conservative treatment. The source of this pain can be difficult to diagnose since the imaging studies that can reveal arthritic changes in or around the facet joints (such as x-ray or MRI) do not do so in all patients. In other words, you could have facet joint inflammation that doesn't appear in your x-ray.

Each facet joint receives its sensory nerve supply one level above and one level below where the nerve branches off the spinal cord. These sensory nerves are known as **medial branch nerves**. Because of these aspects of anatomy, multiple spinal levels need to be injected to achieve the desired effect.

In most cases, up to three facet joint levels are injected on each side at one time. Injections are performed under x-ray guidance to ensure

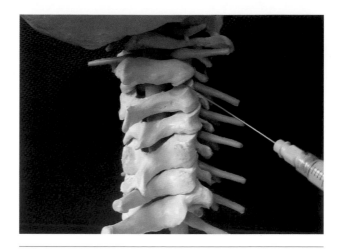

FIGURE 7.4　Typical needle placement for a facet block.

safety and the best effect (figure 7.4). These injections may be given into the facet joint itself or along the medial branch nerve. Generally, a diagnostic facet injection (**facet block**, or medial branch block) is first performed with an anesthetic such as lidocaine to determine which spinal facet level is causing the pain. A positive test would result in significant pain relief for several hours to several days. Steroids may also be added as a therapeutic injection, which could help to extend the effect of the procedure to several weeks. For some people, a series of injections at multiple levels made over several weeks is necessary before the facet joints generating the pain are identified.

Once the pain-generating levels of the spine are identified, the nerves to the facet joints (medial branches) can be deadened in a procedure called *ablation* to provide more long-term relief. Ablation can be done chemically with a substance such as phenol; with heat (**radiofrequency ablation**, also known as **RFA**); or with cold (cryolysis). These procedures are performed in a similar fashion to the facet blocks, under x-ray guidance. They can cause increased pain for a few days after the procedure, but they generally give better long-term relief than do steroid injections. Maximum pain relief may take up to several weeks to occur.

My Neck Hurts!

Radiofrequency ablation is the most common neurolysis (nerve deadening) procedure performed to reduce facet-mediated pain, although it is typically reserved for patients who have failed more conservative treatments. A needle probe is heated along the medial branch nerve, deadening it before it enters the facet joint. Studies have demonstrated that about 50 percent of appropriate patients respond well to this technique, with pain reduction lasting for up to twelve months. There is a small chance that the pain will temporarily worsen rather than improving. Another rare complication specific to facet blocks, or facet nerve ablation, is damage to an unintended nerve or the spinal cord.

■ Teaching Pain a Lesson

As a kindergarten teacher who loved her work, Tonya had always had a high tolerance for noise. Shrieking children, toppling boxes of art supplies, and outbursts of tears didn't faze her. But after being involved in a bad car accident, she found those same sounds almost intolerable.

She was a passenger when another vehicle T-boned the car on the driver's side, and she and the driver knocked heads. Immediately after the accident, Tonya experienced neck and upper back pain and stiffness. She started getting headaches, too. Until then, she had enjoyed good health and an active lifestyle. Now, at age 36, she had "tight and achy muscles all the time in my neck, shoulders, and upper back. On a scale of 1 to 10, my daily pain was a 7, and noise aggravated my pain. I also felt off-balance, the way you do when you're on a ship." But there was more than physical pain to Tonya's ordeal. "I felt moody and down all the time and had difficulty falling and staying asleep."

Episodes of worsening pain sent Tonya to her local emergency room on a regular basis. But x-rays of her neck were normal. Her primary care doctor referred her to a neurologist, who put her on a combination of Topamax, Zanaflex, Naprosyn, and Fioricet and told her "things will get better over time." The drugs eased the pain, but it was still there. She decided to try chiropractic treatment. Although it helped relieve her upper back pain, it made her neck pain and headaches worse.

Some years before, her husband had had lumbar surgery. He asked his neurosurgeon to recommend a pain specialist for Tonya, and that was when she was referred to another neurologist. He placed Tonya on oral steroids for two weeks, which helped resolve the dizziness she was experiencing and reduced the frequency of severe pain episodes. It had no effect, however, on her daily pain. Next, she received trigger point injections with occipital nerve blocks, which significantly decreased her neck, upper back, and head pain for four to six weeks before wearing off. These injections were performed as needed for several months. With subsequent radiofrequency ablation of the occipital nerves, her headaches were greatly reduced.

Tonya's therapy now consists of regular trigger point injections (every four to six weeks) to control her neck pain along with the use of a muscle stimulation unit at home. She also continues to take Topamax and Zanaflex daily and has started a physical therapy program. "I am not pain free, but I'm making steady progress under my treatment plan." Now that her pain is "manageable," she plans to teach again.

"After my accident, I lost my job since I couldn't perform my duties. Although I am nervous about returning to the classroom, where it can be noisy and stressful, I know that my doctor's relentless efforts to decrease my pain will help me get through it."

EPIDURAL INJECTIONS

Injection of steroids around the spinal membrane (dura mater) can be helpful for nerve-related neck pain. The procedure bathes the spinal nerves with steroids to reduce the inflammation that can lead to pain and abnormal sensations. These injections are most helpful for conditions related to nerve root irritation (radiculopathy) such as spinal stenosis or a herniated or ruptured disc (see chapter 2). **Epidural injections** are more commonly used when there is a structural abnormality in the neck that is associated with radiating (radicular) pain, tingling, or numbness into one or both arms. A series of injections is performed over three to six weeks. To avoid any long-term side effects from the steroid, most physicians will not perform more than three series of epidural injections over a one-year period.

Epidural injections are performed under real-time x-ray guidance (fluoroscopy). The area to be injected is cleaned with an iodine solution and then numbed with a local anesthetic. For a *translaminar*, or an *interlaminar*, epidural injection, the needle is inserted between the vertebrae in the lower neck, between the spinous processes. The medication travels up the epidural space to bathe nerve roots higher up in the neck. A *transforaminal* epidural injection, otherwise known as a **selective nerve root block**, can also be performed. This type of epidural injects medication at the level of the specific spinal nerve believed to be causing the symptoms (figure 7.5). Studies have reported improvement in symptoms for up to six months with epidural injections.

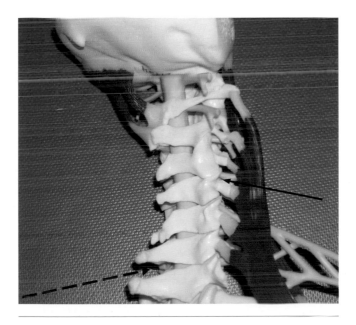

FIGURE 7.5   Needle placement for a translaminar cervical epidural injection is usually between the spinous processes (dashed line); for a transforaminal injection, it is along the nerve root (solid line).

Complications can include bleeding and infection. Rarely, the needle is inserted too far through the dura and into the cerebrospinal fluid. (This is considered an accidental spinal tap.) This is usually not a problem, but if this happens, the steroid cannot be injected. The most common effect from this complication is a headache, due to a slow leak of spinal fluid from the puncture site. In most cases, such a leak will seal itself with time. A needle inserted farther than the cerebrospinal fluid space could penetrate the spinal cord or nerve roots and possibly result in weakness, numbness, or other neurological symptoms. This is highly unlikely when the injections are performed by a skilled physician. Fluoroscopic guidance helps to minimize this possibility.

PROLOTHERAPY

Prolotherapy (proliferative injection therapy) is the use of a chemical irritant injected into tendons or ligaments in an attempt to cause local inflammation. Various chemicals may be injected, including glycerin, phenol (an alcohol), dextrose (a sugar), or cod liver oil extract. The inflammation caused by these substances is thought to secondarily result in new connective tissue growth, strengthening tendons and ligaments and subsequently providing pain relief. Injections are performed in a similar fashion to trigger point injections, without x-ray or any other imaging for guidance. Injections may be performed weekly or monthly, depending on an individual's response to treatment. Because of a lack of controlled studies supporting the effectiveness of prolotherapy, most insurance companies consider it an investigational therapy and will not cover the cost of treatment. It is not widely used by pain specialists in the United States.

ANY INJECTION TREATMENT has risks, including bleeding and infection. Additionally, although slight, there is always the possibility of an allergic reaction any time a foreign substance is injected into the body. If you tend to bruise easily or are taking a blood thinner such as warfarin (Coumadin), notify your physician prior to an injection, as you may be more prone to bleeding. A vasovagal reaction (drop in blood pressure from the experience of the procedure) is also possible (this is true for any injection) and can lead to dizziness, nausea, and even passing out. Serious complications from injection therapy, however, are very rare.

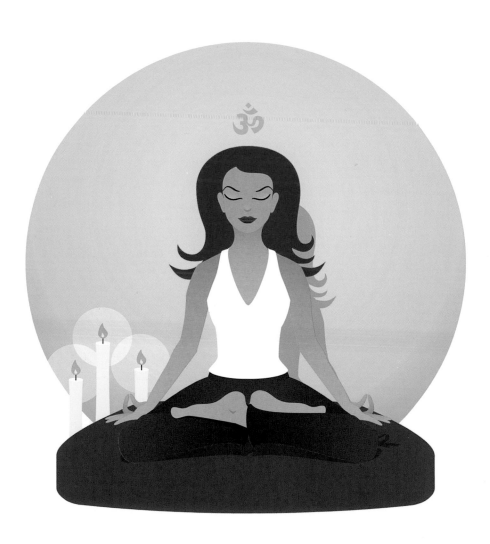

Complementary and Alternative Therapies

Healing the Body, Mind, and Spirit

The mental and emotional effects of chronic pain are well documented. Your medical treatment plan should include a plan for attending to your mental health as well as your physical health. You cannot successfully address chronic pain without taking a complete approach that recognizes the reciprocal mind-body relationship.

There are several so-called complementary and alternative therapies that I recommend, as well as some that I do *not* recommend. I include information on both categories in this chapter because over the years I have found that I spend as much time speaking with my patients about why I *don't* endorse a particular treatment as I do describing the proven ones that I urge them to investigate. The first section of this chapter is devoted to the therapies that are widely acknowledged to be beneficial.

COUNSELING

Mental health professionals have diverse roles and titles. Some specialize in the psychological issues of people with chronic pain. This is why the mental health component of a treatment plan can include a referral to one or more mental health practitioners.

Psychiatrists are physicians (M.D. or D.O.) who after medical school complete a residency in psychiatry. In 1950 there were very few medications available for psychological disorders, but the practice of modern medicine today involves hundreds of FDA-approved medications. Therefore, medical practices and training have become increasingly specialized. Many physicians treating neck pain may be uncomfortable prescribing and monitoring medications for depression, anxiety, and sleep, especially for people with complex mental health disorders. Psychiatrists, on the other hand, have expertise in assessing complex psychological issues and in managing medications that general practitioners may have less experience monitoring.

For people with chronic pain, a referral does not indicate that the referring physician believes the person is "crazy"; it simply means that the treating physician wants the patient to have comprehensive and appropriate care. Most psychiatrists do not engage in extended counseling but instead manage medications and partner with clinical psychologists and counselors to provide counseling services.

Depending on the laws of the state in which you reside, several kinds of mental health providers may be licensed to provide general counseling and pain counseling, including clinical psychologists, counseling psychologists, licensed professional counselors, licensed independent social workers, and religious counselors. Finding the right counselor is similar to finding the right physician. Among professionals with appropriate training, you will want one with whom you can develop a trusting and honest therapeutic relationship. Just as a physician develops a medical treatment plan, a psychologist or counselor will develop a mental health treatment plan. Some aspects of a pain counseling treatment plan may be surprising. In addition to learning relaxation techniques and discussing stress management, some people may need to address and resolve grief associated with a loss of freedom in the ability to perform daily activities as well as the impact of chronic pain on family relationships and functioning, which may mean marriage, partner, or family counseling.

The impact of chronic pain on vocation, education, and relationships varies across an individual's life span; therefore, no two counseling treatment plans are the same. Generally, all plans should address social relationships and the need for continued community involvement, motivation to engage and maintain treatment, and underlying psychological issues that may undermine treatment.

BIOFEEDBACK

Biofeedback provides auditory and visual feedback in real time on specific biological functions, including skin temperature, heart rate, breathing rate, sweating, muscle tension, and brain waves. By providing feedback on these physical reactions, this therapy helps the patient learn how to better control the body's responses to stimuli. For patients with chronic pain, this means reducing tension in specific muscles that are tense or overactive.

During biofeedback treatments, electric wires are attached to the surface of the skin with metal disks or stickers, usually on the head or shoulders (figure 8.1). No needles are involved, and the procedure does not cause discomfort or pain. In fact, most people find biofeedback treatments relaxing and enjoyable.

Biofeedback can be helpful in treating many medical and psycho-

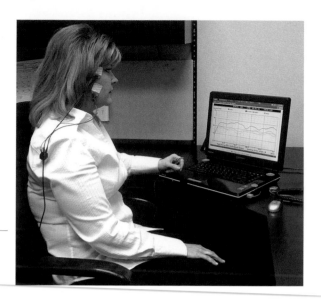

FIGURE 8.1 A patient hooked up to biofeedback equipment.

logical problems, particularly when used in conjunction with other therapies such as medication, counseling, or physical therapy. For those with chronic neck and upper back pain, biofeedback treatment using electromyography (EMG) may be the most useful. In this technique, electrodes can be placed on the painful muscles, most commonly over the trapezus or semispinalis muscles. The electrodes are connected to a computer that helps the person see and hear a representation of baseline and contracted muscle activity in these painful areas. Specific relaxation techniques—breathing and meditation or guided imagery—are taught, and with practice, the person is able to quiet activity in the neck muscles. Once this technique is mastered, it can be practiced daily at home to prevent or to treat muscle spasm and pain. It can also help ease insomnia, which is associated with chronic pain.

ACUPUNCTURE

Traditional Chinese medicine teaches that more than 2,000 points in the body connect with pathways, or **meridians**, that conduct energy, known as **Qi** (pronounced "chee"). These points are believed to have greater concentrations of sensory nerve endings and blood vessels than the surrounding tissue. The aim of acupuncture treatment is to correct any imbalance in Qi by stimulating these points with the insertion of fine needles, and thereby "clearing" any blockages to the flow of energy. Modern science suggests that other mechanisms for acupuncture's effectiveness include the release of endorphins and other pain-reducing substances produced by the body. Acupuncture may also act as sensory distraction to pain. In the hands of a skilled practitioner, acupuncture is relatively painless, and the chance of infection or bleeding is low.

Very thin, disposable stainless-steel needles are inserted and then twisted into the skin in a particular pattern along the meridians (figure 8.2). The site of needle placement and the number of needles is determined by the individual's symptoms (figure 8.3). The needles are usually left in the skin for 30 to 40 minutes. Some people report a small pricking sensation along with an ache, numbness, and warmth in the area of the needle. Some feel relaxed after the treatment, while others feel energized. Five to seven treatments may be given over three to eight weeks for a complete treatment regimen.

Some practitioners apply an electric current to the needles, which may increase the effectiveness of the treatment; however, improper technique or excessive electrical stimulation can cause temporary tissue achiness. In 1997, the National Institutes of Health issued a consensus statement regarding the clinical effects of acupuncture: based on studies, clear evidence had demonstrated the effectiveness of acupuncture in the treatment of

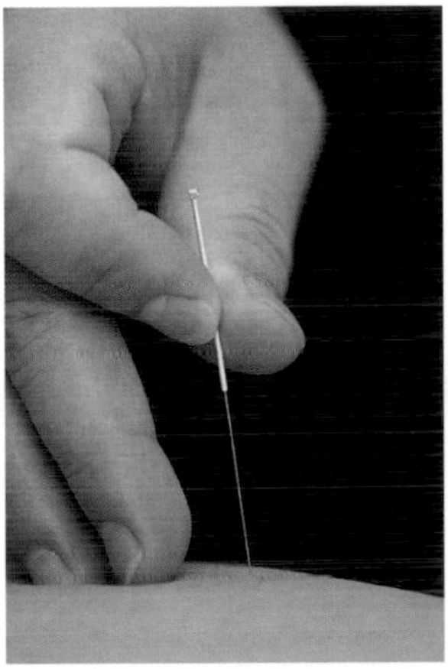

FIGURE 8.2 Acupuncture needle being inserted into the skin. Image courtesy of StockXpert. Used by permission.

Complementary and Alternative Therapies

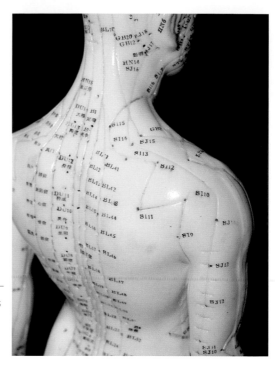

FIGURE 8.3 A map of numerous acupuncture points in the neck and upper back. Image courtesy of StockXpert. Used by permission.

postsurgical and chemotherapy-related nausea and vomiting, as well as for postsurgical dental pain. The verdict is not in for the treatment of other pain syndromes, and clinical trials have shown mixed results. For neck pain specifically, some studies have reported a more than 50 percent reduction in neck pain after acupuncture compared with a placebo treatment, while others have shown no benefit. Further research is needed to determine whether acupuncture should be recommended as a worthwhile option for chronic neck pain.

Most states regulate the practice of acupuncture with certification and training requirements. Practitioners with qualifications include allopathic (M.D.) physicians, osteopathic (D.O.) physicians, chiropractors, dentists, and traditional Chinese acupuncturists. Acupuncture treatments are not covered by insurance in most instances, and the quality of trained practitioners may vary greatly in a particular area. Despite having to pay cash for the procedure, more than one million Americans receive acupuncture yearly.

My Neck Hurts!

YOGA

Yoga is an ancient practice that originated in India over 4,000 years ago. It combines physical exercise and stretching with breathing and meditation techniques. Some people feel that the process of yoga represents the ultimate in the mind-body connection. When performed properly and regularly, it can reduce pain by increasing flexibility and by lessening stress and tension that commonly trigger pain.

The stretches performed in yoga with regulated breathing and meditation can reduce pain in a manner similar to what takes place in biofeedback. Beginners or those who are not flexible can still benefit from yoga. *A cautionary note: some yoga techniques should not be performed by anyone with significant spinal disease.*

A generation ago, yoga was considered a fringe activity. Today organizations as mainstream as YMCAs, senior centers, and hospitals offer regular classes. There has been a groundswell of interest. According to a 2002 survey by the National Center for Health Statistics, more than 10 million Americans practice yoga; 21 percent reported using it specifically for neck or back pain, although the effectiveness of this therapy was not assessed in the survey. While some scientific studies have suggested that yoga is helpful for low back pain, no known studies have been performed on patients specifically with neck pain.

Advocates of yoga believe it helps achieve harmony between the mind and body. It does so using specific physical and mental practices:

- Proper breathing is used to achieve optimal oxygen intake through slow, rhythmic, deep breaths with a pause between breaths. This exercise is meant to increase mental focus as well as physical energy. Each movement should be guided by coordinated breathing.
- Proper relaxation is used to attain a sense of mental calm so that the body can release muscular tension.
- Proper exercise, because the physical body is meant to move and

exercise regularly, involves using the yoga postures to stretch and tone the muscles and increase blood flow.

- Proper diet helps maintain a healthy mental state and spiritual awareness. A proper diet of natural foods nourishes both the body and the mind. Eating should be done only in moderation to keep the body light and the mind calm.
- Positive thinking and meditation help remove negative thoughts and maintain a peaceful mind.

Although there are many different forms of yoga, they all use these common guiding principles. The following figures (8.4–8.6) are examples of classic yoga postures.

FIGURE 8.4   Sukhasana is a starting position that helps focus awareness on breathing, body posture, and sensations. © 2006 Darren Green. Image from BigStockPhoto.com.

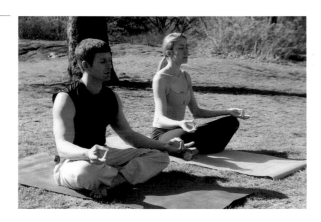

FIGURE 8.5   The modified child's pose (bala-asana) stretches and strengthens the shoulders and the cervical and lumbar areas of the spine. © 2006 Darren Green. Image from BigStockPhoto .com.

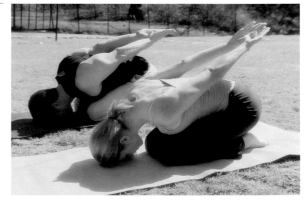

My Neck Hurts!

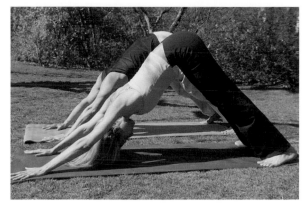

FIGURE 8.6 Downward-facing dog (adho mukha svanasana) builds strength and flexibility in the spine and hamstrings. © 2006 Darren Green. Image from BigStockPhoto.com.

PILATES

Pilates is an exercise program named after its originator, Joseph Pilates, that has been around since the early 1900s. It is based on maintaining proper body alignment while stretching and strengthening the muscles in a series of no-impact movements performed on a floor mat or on specially designed platforms or bars equipped with resistance bands and pulleys.

Pilates' inspiration came from his own physical limitations early in life. As a young child, he suffered from rickets. In an attempt to strengthen his frail body, he became interested in body conditioning. Studying various methods of exercise and fitness, he gradually developed his own philosophy and a method of exercise that he called "Contrology." His initial approach used a system of springs for resistance, an idea that led eventually to the development of equipment he designed to help disabled and immobilized soldiers in World War I. When Pilates moved from Europe to the United States in 1925, he brought his unique exercise system with him, and it quickly became popular with professional dancers and athletes. In the 1980s, Pilates classes became the workout of choice for Hollywood celebrities, and, not surprisingly, soon after it became widely sought by the general public.

A few basic principles govern how Pilates is performed:

1. Maintain a neutral spinal posture while performing exercises.
2. Use precise breathing to promote mental focus and centering.
3. Develop concentration for maximum muscle efficiency and control.
4. Develop the low back and abdominal muscles to aid in maintaining spinal alignment.
5. Increase muscle tone, strength, and flexibility.

The most commonly used piece of Pilates equipment today is the Reformer (figure 8.7). This device consists of a rolling platform that is secured at one end with springs. Resistance is produced by pushing off the frame of the device, or by pulling on ropes, with the arms or legs.

The Wunda Chair is a platform in the form of a bench with a horizontal bar that is attached to springs. Resistance is produced by pushing on the bar while sitting on or in front of the chair.

Pilates exercises that can be performed without the use of equipment are known as mat exercises, which are a series performed on a thin, nonslip floor mat (figure 8.8). This type of Pilates is more often performed in small groups. The same principles of keeping the spine

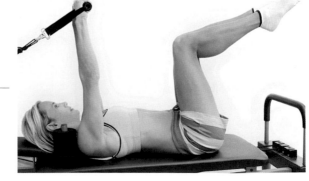

FIGURE 8.7   Demonstration using a Pilates Reformer. © 2005 Nicholas Sutcliffe. Image from BigStockPhoto.com.

My Neck Hurts!

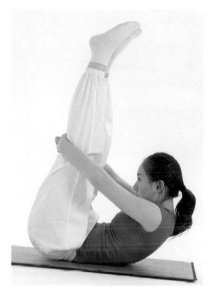

FIGURE 8.8 A Pilates mat exercise used to improve flexibility © 2005 JinYoung Lee. Image from BigStockPhoto.com.

in a neutral position, and regulating one's breathing, are applied to this type of Pilates.

Pilates may be most helpful for patients with only mild to moderately severe pain or those who are trying to improve strength and prevent relapse after recovery. The potential benefits can extend to improved posture and a better awareness of muscle tension and its relationship to pain. The frequency of sessions can vary greatly depending on the person's motivation and ability to attend classes, from once to several times per week. This type of program is not for everyone, because it can be physically and mentally challenging and takes significant personal commitment to succeed.

OTHER COMPLEMENTARY AND ALTERNATIVE THERAPIES

There are a multitude of other nontraditional, or alternative, therapies that are not discussed in detail here. Most of these therapies have no significant literature to support their use in the treatment of chronic

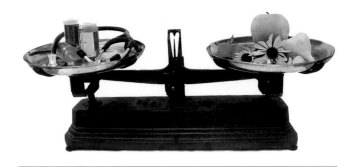

FIGURE 8.9   Keeping the different aspects of life in balance is a goal of many complementary therapies. © 2005 Gordon Swanson. Image from BigStockPhoto.com.

neck pain. Some of these practices, however, are similar to alternative treatments previously described and may be helpful. These include **acupressure, Alexander technique, Feldenkrais method, Rolfing**, and **Tai Chi**.

Acupressure is based on a premise similar to acupuncture: that the body's energy force (or Qi) flows through meridian pathways. Instead of using a needle as in acupuncture, the practitioner applies pressure with his or her hands to specific points along the meridian to restore a normal healthy energy flow.

The Alexander technique was invented by the Austrian teacher and actor Matthias Alexander. He developed a method to make people become more aware of their bodies and balance their postures. Originally designed as a lesson to help his voice students, this technique evolved into a system of rebalancing the body by breathing while maintaining correct posture and movements in an attempt to improve physical and emotional well-being. Alexander treatment is not unlike other alternative techniques such as yoga and biofeedback.

The Feldenkrais method was developed by the Israeli physicist Moshe Feldenkrais. He developed a method of healthy movements and breathing to improve self-awareness after his own personal experience with sports injuries. The goals of this method include increasing range

My Neck Hurts!

of motion, flexibility, and coordination. Practitioners generally do not diagnose or treat illness. Rather they teach by "awareness through movement" lessons. The practitioner verbally guides a student through a sequence of movements, or "functional integration," in which the student's movements are fine-tuned through light touch. Sessions are 30 to 60 minutes in length, and there are hundreds of lessons to choose from. Training for practitioners includes over 800 hours of instruction over a three- to four-year period for certification through the Feldenkrais Guild of North America. Feldenkrais teachers are neither regulated nor licensed by state medical boards.

Rolfing (structural integration) is a method of deep tissue massage developed by the biochemist Ida Rolf, Ph.D. This manual therapy seeks to separate any bound connective tissue (fascia) and to allow this tissue to move more freely. A Rolfing program generally involves ten one-hour sessions with a specific goal for each session. Rolfing claims to align and lengthen the body through these treatments. No studies have evaluated Rolfing for neck or upper back pain.

Tai Chi is a Chinese practice somewhat similar to yoga and other mind-body therapies (figure 8.10). The goal of Tai Chi is to balance the two opposing life forces yin and yang and thus create harmony between the mind and body. Some studies suggest that performing Tai Chi regularly can improve cardiovascular health, strength, and coordina-

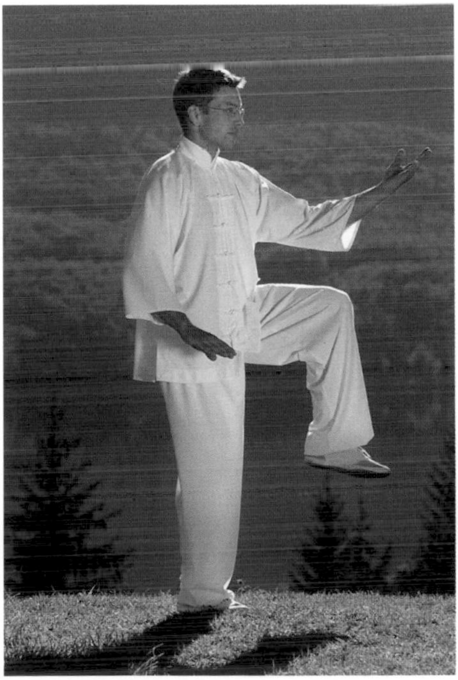

FIGURE 8.10   A Tai Chi pose. © 2006 Simon Krzic. Image from BigStockPhoto.com.

Complementary and Alternative Therapies   133

tion. Reducing tension and creating a sense of well-being may also be achieved with practice. No studies have demonstrated improvement of neck and upper back pain symptoms specifically.

As stated at the beginning of this chapter, some therapies are *not* recommended here because, at best, these treatments have no clinical effect on pain, although a placebo effect is certainly possible. At worst, they can be potentially harmful. Alternatives that I do *not* recommend as effective in the treatment of chronic neck pain include **aromatherapy, chelation therapy, craniosacral therapy, herbal therapy, homeopathy, magnet therapy, reflexology, Reiki**, and **therapeutic touch**.

Aromatherapy involves essential oils extracted from plants and flowers that are applied or massaged into the skin, inhaled, or added to bathwater. An aromatherapist may recommend a certain aroma to treat a specific medical condition. Using aromas can aid in relaxation, but there is no evidence that it is helpful in the treatment of neck and upper back pain.

Chelation therapy is a series of intravenous infusions containing organic chemical ethylenediaminetetraacetic acid (EDTA) or various other substances. EDTA is a water-soluble substance that binds multiple metal ions and has legitimate uses in people whose bodies contain toxic levels of heavy metals, such as lead, mercury, copper, or cadmium. Heavy metal toxicity, however, is very rare. Advocates of chelation therapy claim positive effects on multiple health problems. An average of twenty to forty intravenous treatments are performed to treat various medical conditions and are not covered by insurance. There is no significant research to suggest this therapy is beneficial in the treatment of neck and upper back pain.

Craniosacral therapy is a nontraditional osteopathic technique developed by William G. Sutherland, D.O., in the 1930s and later promoted by John Upledger, D.O., in the 1980s. Craniosacral therapy is a controversial concept within the osteopathic community, but despite this controversy, it is used by many other practitioners, including chiropractors, dentists, physical therapists, and massage therapists.

The technique is based on the belief that there is a natural rhythm of the fluid (cerebrospinal fluid) surrounding the brain and spinal cord that can be felt. This pulsation is reported to normally occur at 10 to 14 cycles per minute and is unrelated to respiration or pulse. Manipulation of the bones of the skull and the meninges (the membranes covering the brain) through gentle touch is thought to balance this rhythm and restore health. Its claims include relief of headaches and neck pain.

There may well be a natural rhythm to the cerebrospinal fluid, but no objective technique has been devised to support this theory. The premise that such a presumed rhythm could be manually manipulated is therefore not supported by the medical literature. There are no studies to suggest that it is a viable treatment for chronic neck and upper back pain, although it is unlikely to be harmful. The treatments are reported to be calming, which is most likely the effect of the practitioner's personal touch, influencing the way a patient feels.

Herbal medicine involves the use of plants or plant extracts to treat disease and promote health. Herbal preparations may include the stem, leaf, flower, root, bark, or fruit of a plant. Many ancient societies used herbs as medical treatment before the age of modern medicine. Significant refinements have occurred in the twentieth century with the advent of preparations in capsule or tablet form. These refinements have allowed for easier usage and some standardization of dosage, which has led to a significant rise in the use of herbs.

Any herb may contain one or more active chemical molecules that have a specific action on the body, but many of the active ingredients may be unknown. The action of these compounds could have positive or negative clinical effects, depending on the properties of the compound and the dosage taken. Examples of chemicals derived from plants in modern medicine include aspirin (originally extracted from the bark of the willow tree) and digitalis (a medicine made from the foxglove plant, used for heart failure). Many other modern medicines have been derived from plant extracts or are synthesized versions of an active plant compound.

Herbal preparations in their natural forms are not regulated by the FDA. Because of this, there is less government oversight regarding potential side effects or claims made by the companies that produce herbs. For these reasons, I urge my patients to exercise caution in using herbal preparations. Rigorous scientific studies are not performed on most herbal preparations to evaluate their clinical effects or potential short-term and long-term side effects. In addition, the potential interactions of herbs with other herbs and prescription medications can be dangerous.

Certain herbs, despite being "natural," have been linked to serious side effects. For example, comfrey and kava have been shown to be associated with liver damage. Also, there is no regulatory guarantee that an herbal preparation does not contain unwanted substances, including metals or microorganisms.

Homeopathy is an alternative discipline based on the concept of "like cures like." Samuel Hahnemann (a German physician) first developed this concept and used the term homeopathy in the early 1800s. Substances that would actually cause a condition or symptom are used in an extremely diluted form to treat that condition or symptom. Multiple dilutions are performed by a process called *dynamization,* or *potentization,* in which the preparation is shaken between dilutions. This concept is completely counterintuitive to the laws of biochemistry and pharmacology on which mainstream medicine is based. Preparations may include various ingredients, including plant extracts, minerals, and even poisons or venoms from animals. The substances are typically mixed in an alcohol or water solution, and very small amounts are taken orally.

In 2005, an in-depth article was published in the *Lancet* that reviewed 110 placebo-controlled trials on homeopathy. The conclusion of this review was that any potential effect of homeopathy was from a placebo effect. Homeopathic preparations are not regulated by the FDA.

Homeopathic practitioners can diagnosis and treat medical conditions by dispensing homeopathic preparations. Depending on the state, these practitioners may include allopathic or osteopathic physicians, naturopathic doctors, dentists, and chiropractors.

Magnet therapy is a self-treatment using small magnets placed on the skin in various locations. This includes the use of necklaces, bracelets, shoe inserts, and patches. Many claims have been made regarding the effects of magnets, including increased blood circulation and reduced inflammation, as well as reduced chronic pain. These claims are not supported by the bulk of scientific evidence. One study by Baylor University in Houston suggests that there may be a positive effect specifically for patients with chronic pain related to previous polio, but the results of this limited study have not been replicated. Other studies have not supported a positive effect in the treatment of other painful conditions, such as low back pain and heel pain. There are no significant studies supporting the use of magnets placed on the skin as a reasonable treatment for neck and upper back pain. No studies have suggested that magnet therapy is harmful (except, possibly, to your checkbook), but magnets should *not* be used in patients with implanted devices such as a pacemaker, vagus nerve stimulator, or spinal cord stimulator, because these devices could be temporarily deactivated by a magnet.

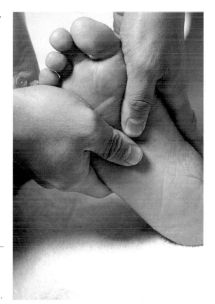

Reflexology, also known as zone therapy, is essentially a massage-like technique for the feet and hands (figure 8.11). This therapy is based on the belief that each organ and part of the

FIGURE 8.11   Reflexology focuses on massage-like manipulation of the feet. © 2006 Suprijono Suharjoto. Image from BigStockPhoto.com.

body is represented by regions in the hands and feet. Proponents of this treatment claim that it can cleanse the body of toxins, increase circulation, improve the health of organs, and balance the body's energy to promote healing. No formal training is required to practice reflexology, and no state or federal body regulates its practice. Although this type of treatment may be relaxing, there is no evidence that the body's regions or organs are connected to specific areas of the feet and hands, and no suggestion that this therapy is effective for neck and upper back pain.

Reiki is a technique that claims to heal through the manipulation of the body's Ki, which means spirit in Japanese, and is similar to the Chinese Qi. It is one of several types of energy therapy. Practitioners of Reiki believe that they can channel or increase the positive Ki and decrease negative energy to heal. The treatments are performed by moving the hands over or slightly touching the patient's body in twelve to fifteen different positions. There is no scientific evidence that such an energy pattern is present or can be manipulated.

Therapeutic touch was developed by a nurse, Dolores Kreiger, R.N., Ph.D., and the natural healer named Dora Kunz. It is a type of energy therapy similar to Reiki. A practitioner manipulates or balances the patient's energy field in order to allow the body to heal. Surprisingly, despite its nonscientific basis, it is most commonly practiced by nurses in a hospital setting. The treatment is performed by the practitioner positioning her hands above or around an individual in an attempt to correct any imbalance in his or her energy field. Each treatment involves four basic steps: calming the patient's mind (centering), evaluating his or her energy field (assessing), correcting any imbalance in the energy field (intervention), and closure. A session may take up to thirty minutes.

There is no certification for therapeutic touch practitioners. As with other energy therapies, there is no scientific basis to the treatment. Despite this, some studies have suggested that therapeutic touch may be helpful in treating some pain, such as fibromyalgia, arthritis, and musculoskeletal pain. These studies, however, were either too small to yield significant results or poorly designed scientifically. The results of an important and carefully constructed trial, published in the *Journal of the American Medical Association* in 1998, disputes the claim of therapeutic touch practitioners that energy fields can be reliably sensed at all.

AS PART OF A PLAN to address chronic pain, complementary and alternative therapies are meant to supplement the medical strategies you and your doctor have developed. Many of these treatments can play an ongoing role in your improved mobility and pain reduction and may even become an essential activity in your daily life.

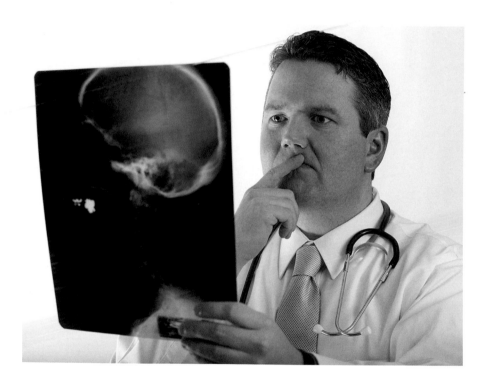

Putting It All Together

The more you know about the various causes of chronic neck pain, the more useful your conversations with your doctor will be in terms of discussing treatment options for alleviating or eliminating the pain. The more you can contribute to the conversation, the better your results will be.

CONTRIBUTING FACTORS IN NECK PAIN

Many factors can play a role in your chronic neck pain. An injury or repetitive strain often starts the pain, which can be further complicated by emotional or social factors.

Your neck pain may not have one obvious cause, so it is important to undergo testing to obtain as much information as possible. At the same time, remember that just because abnormalities are seen on an x-ray or MRI scan (such as disc disease or arthritic bone thickening), that does not necessarily explain why you are having pain. Understanding and accepting that one single physical

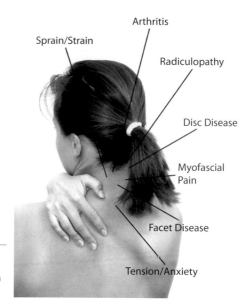

Arthritis

Sprain/Strain

Radiculopathy

Disc Disease

Myofascial
Pain

Facet Disease

Tension/Anxiety

FIGURE 9.1   Common influences on
neck and upper back pain. © 2009 Martin
Novak. Image from BigStockPhoto.com.

abnormality may not be the reason for the pain is important when talking to your doctor about expectations for improvement and options for treatment (figure 9.1).

THE CYCLE OF PAIN

No medical problem occurs in isolation from your social and emotional health, and neck pain is no exception. Tension, anxiety, and depression can play a role in the onset or continuation of chronic pain. When pain continues for a long time, it can lead to depression and even feelings of despair. This in turn commonly results in nonrestful sleep and generalized fatigue, which can worsen the underlying pain. This leads to a cycle of pain (figure 9.2). Developing and following a treatment plan that addresses emotional or mental as well as physical factors is essential to breaking this cycle.

Before your first appointment with a physician who specializes

My Neck Hurts!

in addressing chronic neck pain, take the time to put together some detailed information about your condition, level of pain, and medical history. This information will be a great help to the doctor—and to you. I offer the questionnaire reproduced on pages 150–53 to my own patients; you can photocopy it or visit my Web site at www.neckpaincare.com (see Neck Pain Questionnaire) and print a copy to fill out before your first appointment.

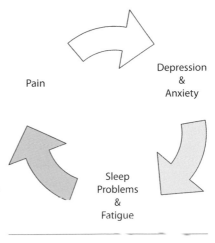

FIGURE 9.2   The cycle of pain and contributing factors.

KNOW YOUR OPTIONS

Most people will start treating their neck pain with simple self-directed treatments using over-the-counter medications, creams or lotions, and heat or ice. When seeking medical help for neck pain, most people will first see their primary care doctor (family physician or internist) or a chiropractor. As with any practitioner, the background and experience of each doctor can vary quite a bit when it comes to understanding the causes, diagnostic tools, and treatment options for neck and upper back pain. You may be surprised at how many physicians are not aware of or do not understand the concepts and options discussed in this book. In addition, doctors are human and therefore may have a bias toward (or against) a particular type of practitioner or treatment type. This is why you, the person seeking treatment, needs to be aware of your choices.

Chapters 3 through 8 cover the multitude of medically accepted nonsurgical therapies that have helped many thousands of people suffering from chronic neck or upper back pain. I have arranged the chap-

TABLE 9.1
Treatment options for neck and upper back pain

Physical and psychological treatments and therapies	Medications	Injections / invasive procedures
Physical therapy, aquatherapy	NSAIDs	Trigger point injections
Cervical traction	Muscle relaxants	Botulinum toxin injections
Heat, ice, ultrasound	Opioids	Epidural injections
TENS, muscle stimulation, PNT	Oral steroids	Facet / medial branch blocks or denervation
OMT, chiropractic, massage	Antidepressants	Occipital nerve blocks
Biofeedback, counseling	Antiseizure medicines	Spinal cord stimulation
Acupuncture, yoga, Pilates	Topical patches or creams	Prolotherapy

ters in the order in which most patients like to approach treatment—and which I usually recommend: from the least invasive or aggressive to the most. Where you begin is a highly personal choice and will depend on many factors, including your diagnosis, your lifestyle, and your threshold for pain.

Tables 9.1 and 9.2 are included as helpful references to turn to after you and your physician have discussed treatment options. Table 9.1 gives an overview of most treatment options available by treatment type, and table 9.2 compares how invasive each option is in comparison to others.

CHOOSING A DOCTOR

Many primary care physicians will refer a patient with neck pain to a neurosurgeon or orthopedic spine surgeon for surgical intervention *before* considering other, minimally or moderately invasive treatments. I believe this is largely due to a lack of knowledge by many physicians about when surgery really needs to be considered. As I tell my patients, "Surgeons do surgery!" Typically, surgeons do not look for opportunities to treat neck pain nonsurgically. You or a family member

TABLE 9.2
Comparison of treatment invasiveness for different levels of pain

	Mild pain	Moderate pain	Severe pain
Noninvasive	Physical therapy, aquatherapy, heat, ice, ultrasound, cervical traction, NSAIDs, muscle relaxants, massage, yoga, Pilates, topical patches or creams	Cervical traction, oral steroids, anti-depressants, anti-seizure medicines, biofeedback, counsel-ing, topical patches or creams	Opioids, anti-depressants, anti-seizure medicines, biofeedback, counseling
Minimally invasive	OMT, chiropractic, TENS, muscle stimulation	PNT, acupuncture, trigger point injec-tions, botulinum toxin injections, occipital nerve blocks	PNT, botulinum toxin injections, prolotherapy, occipital nerve blocks
Invasive		Epidural injections, facet/medial branch blocks or denervation	Epidural injections, facet/medial branch blocks or denerva-tion, spinal cord stimulation

may have already consulted with a surgeon and be familiar with this bias.

But as this book describes, a small disc bulge or arthritis shown on an x-ray or MRI report doesn't mean that the mild abnormality is the cause of or even a significant contributor to your pain. If it is deter-mined that surgery is not necessary or appropriate, then what? This can be a confusing time for a patient, especially when there is a great desire to find a clear reason for the pain and "fix it" immediately. There are medical experts who can help you.

If your primary care doctor does not initially recommend that you see a specialist with more extensive expertise in treating neck pain, you should ask for a referral. Such specialists include anesthesiolo-gists (pain specialists), **physiatrists** (rehabilitation doctors), and neurologists.

- Anesthesiologists (M.D. or D.O.) are trained initially to perform procedures related to anesthesia for surgeries. Some of these doctors train an extra year to learn how to treat patients with chronic pain. They may be more often referred to as "pain specialists" than a neurologist or physiatrist is, even though the latter treat pain as well. The title "pain specialist" is particularly appropriate if the physician has obtained additional training in the treatment of pain and has passed a test to become board certified in pain management.

  Board certification is not required to treat patients with pain, nor does it mean that the particular practitioner is competent. It does mean that he or she has completed a specific course of study in pain treatment and passed a test on the subject. Anesthesiologists' bias may be toward performing invasive procedures because this is what they have been primarily trained to do.

- Physiatrists (physical medicine and rehabilitation specialists) also care for patients with chronic neck and upper back pain. These doctors (whether M.D. or D.O.) have special training in the diagnosis and treatment of diseases of the muscles, peripheral nerves, and musculoskeletal system. Their background stresses an understanding of the mechanical nature of neck pain and the issues involved in rehabilitation after injury of the spine or surrounding structures. They may also aid in diagnosis by performing an EMG (electromyography) or by ordering further testing. Some physiatrists obtain additional training to learn how to perform spinal injections such as epidurals or facet blocks. These doctors are known as *interventionalists*.

- Neurologists (M.D. or D.O.) have extensive training in diseases of the brain, spinal cord, and peripheral nerves. Their training stresses the involvement of the nervous system in chronic pain. They tend to have more experience and understanding in the treatment of headaches commonly associated with neck pain. Because of this understanding of the nervous system, they can aid in diagnosis only using a procedure such as EMG and they can be involved in treatment. Neurologists may use antiseizure medications to treat pain more often than other physicians because of their extensive experience with these drugs. They are more likely than other physicians to treat a patient with a fairly conservative plan because they are less likely to be trained in the use of spinal injections.

Because of these differences in specialist training and philosophy, a single practitioner may not provide all treatment options mentioned in this book. This is especially true when it comes to opioid (narcotic) medications. Many doctors do not prescribe these drugs because of the potential for abuse and the need for close monitoring. Other practitioners who provide conservative care include physical therapists, chiropractors, and massage therapists.

After an initial consultation, the extent and type of testing performed (such as x-ray, MRI) may depend on the practitioner's examination findings as well as the severity and length of the pain syndrome you are experiencing. Your primary care doctor will probably have an established referral pattern to certain doctors in your community for the treatment of neck and upper back pain. This physician preference is usually based on his or her positive experience with a particular specialist, but you should always ask why a physician is being recommended. The type of physician is not necessarily as important as his or her reputation in the community, skill set, and ability to relate to patients. The referring physician should be able to discuss these points with you.

Each time a specialist sees you for a visit, a note is sent to your primary doctor to update him or her on your progress or to detail any problems or side effects from treatment. This continuity and communication is imperative for comprehensive care.

If you eventually decide to consider spinal surgery as an option for treatment, you will need to consult with an **orthopedic surgeon** or **neurosurgeon**. Orthopedic surgeons (M.D. or D.O.) are initially trained in the surgical and nonsurgical treatment of diseases of the joints and musculoskeletal system. Some opt for subsequent education to perform spinal surgery. Neurosurgeons (M.D. or D.O.) are trained to perform both brain and spinal surgery. I believe that the local reputation and skill level of the surgeon are more important than the type.

Surgeons will provide an opinion about whether intervention is needed or appropriate, but they will not provide long-term care of patients with neck pain. After surgery, limited treatment may be continued for six to twelve months, including postsurgical pain medications and physical therapy for rehabilitation. If further pain care is needed, the patient is normally referred back to the primary care doctor or to a pain specialist.

■ When Your Job Is a Pain in the Neck

Matthew had always taken pride in his above-average physical strength and endurance. "I could never see myself working at a desk job." His job as a welder was demanding, but he enjoyed it, and even at age 52 he had an edge on his younger co-workers. Twenty years of experience had given him skills they had yet to acquire.

He had become accustomed to neck pain at the end of the workday and treated it with over-the-counter drugs such as Motrin and Tylenol. But about four years ago, his pain became constant and more severe, including new symptoms of right-side weakness and numbness. His primary care doctor ordered x-rays and an MRI of his neck, which revealed severe degenerative disc disease with associated arthritis, and a herniated disc between the fifth and sixth cervical vertebrae that was pressing on the C6 nerve on the right side. An EMG confirmed that the C6 nerve was being actively damaged.

Matthew was referred to an orthopedic spine surgeon, who recommended surgery; Matthew agreed and soon after underwent a fusion with a plate and screws. "The numbness in my arm was gone immediately after surgery. With physical therapy, I started to get my strength back, but I still had a lot of neck pain." This is when he was referred to an anesthesiologist who specialized in treating chronic pain.

The specialist's evaluation indicated that most of Matthew's pain was coming from his facet joints. As the doctor explained, wearing a heavy welding helmet for years and popping his head forward to flip his mask down had caused severe facet trauma. He recommended diagnostic facet injections and prescribed Vicodin for breakthrough pain as well as the daily use of Flector patches.

Two rounds of facet injections provided significant relief for up to two weeks each time. Radiofrequency ablations were subsequently performed to the facet nerves, finally giving Matthew long-term pain relief. Although he still has pain once or twice a week, he has found that Vicodin addresses that, and no daily treatment or medications are needed. "I'm more careful now and flip my mask with my hand. It was a hard habit to break, but I'm just glad I'm still able to do my job."

LIVING WITH CHRONIC PAIN does not have to be your fate. By understanding more about what's causing your pain, both physically and mentally, and investigating the many treatment choices available, you can become an informed decision maker. With the help of the right medical professional, you can address the pain and improve the quality of your life.

Neck Pain Questionnaire

Patient name: _____   Date seen: _____

Birth date: _____   Age: _____   Sex: Male   Female

Please answer the following questions regarding your neck pain.

A. Neck pain onset
1. My neck pain started _____ years ago at _____ years of age.
2. Any associated trauma or injury?   Yes/No
   Explain: _____
3. Loss of Consciousness?   Yes/No
4. Any history of infection around your brain or spinal cord?   Yes/No

B. Current neck pain frequency
1. My neck pain occurs _____ all the time **or** _____ times per day / week / month.
2. Has the frequency recently changed?   Yes/No
   Comments: _____

C. Neck pain location (circle any that apply)
Right side   Left side   Both sides
Shoulders   Upper back   Back of the head
Other: _____

D. Neck pain quality (circle any that apply)
Throbbing   Pulsating   Nagging
Pressure   Squeezing   Bandlike
Stabbing   Sharp   Aching
Dull
Comments: _____

E. Neck pain timing (circle any that apply)
My neck pain tends to occur: when I wake up   in the morning   in the afternoon
                               after work   in the evening   during sleep
Comments: _____

F. Neck pain duration:
On the days that my neck pain is present, it lasts:
☐ all day
☐ 2–6 hours
☐ 6–12 hours
☐ 12–18 hours

My Neck Hurts!

G. Neck pain severity (circle the average pain level)

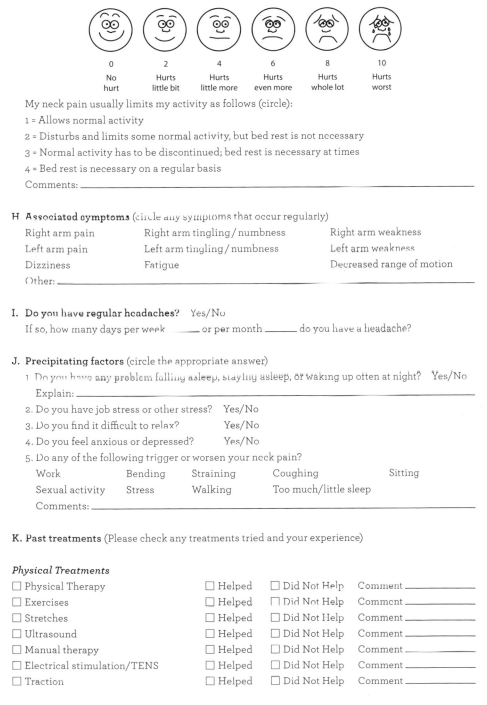

0	2	4	6	8	10
No hurt	Hurts little bit	Hurts little more	Hurts even more	Hurts whole lot	Hurts worst

My neck pain usually limits my activity as follows (circle):

1 = Allows normal activity

2 = Disturbs and limits some normal activity, but bed rest is not necessary

3 = Normal activity has to be discontinued; bed rest is necessary at times

4 = Bed rest is necessary on a regular basis

Comments: _____

H Associated symptoms (circle any symptoms that occur regularly)

Right arm pain	Right arm tingling/numbness	Right arm weakness
Left arm pain	Left arm tingling/numbness	Left arm weakness
Dizziness	Fatigue	Decreased range of motion

Other: _____

I. Do you have regular headaches?   Yes/No

If so, how many days per week _____ or per month _____ do you have a headache?

J. Precipitating factors (circle the appropriate answer)

1 Do you have any problem falling asleep, staying asleep, or waking up often at night?   Yes/No

Explain: _____

2. Do you have job stress or other stress?   Yes/No

3. Do you find it difficult to relax?   Yes/No

4. Do you feel anxious or depressed?   Yes/No

5. Do any of the following trigger or worsen your neck pain?

Work	Bending	Straining	Coughing	Sitting
Sexual activity	Stress	Walking	Too much/little sleep	

Comments: _____

K. Past treatments (Please check any treatments tried and your experience)

Physical Treatments

☐ Physical Therapy	☐ Helped	☐ Did Not Help	Comment _____
☐ Exercises	☐ Helped	☐ Did Not Help	Comment _____
☐ Stretches	☐ Helped	☐ Did Not Help	Comment _____
☐ Ultrasound	☐ Helped	☐ Did Not Help	Comment _____
☐ Manual therapy	☐ Helped	☐ Did Not Help	Comment _____
☐ Electrical stimulation/TENS	☐ Helped	☐ Did Not Help	Comment _____
☐ Traction	☐ Helped	☐ Did Not Help	Comment _____

Putting It All Together

☐ OMT (Osteopathic manipulation therapy)	☐ Helped	☐ Did Not Help	Comment _____
☐ Chiropractic	☐ Helped	☐ Did Not Help	Comment _____
☐ Massage	☐ Helped	☐ Did Not Help	Comment _____
☐ Home traction	☐ Helped	☐ Did Not Help	Comment _____
☐ Home electrical stimulation/TENS	☐ Helped	☐ Did Not Help	Comment _____
☐ PNT/PENS	☐ Helped	☐ Did Not Help	Comment _____
☐ Acupuncture/acupressure	☐ Helped	☐ Did Not Help	Comment _____
☐ Lidoderm patches	☐ Helped	☐ Did Not Help	Comment _____
☐ Flector patches	☐ Helped	☐ Did Not Help	Comment _____
☐ Biofeedback/pain counseling	☐ Helped	☐ Did Not Help	Comment _____
☐ Other _____	☐ Helped	☐ Did Not Help	Comment _____

Medications

☐ Tylenol/acetaminophen	☐ Helped	☐ Did Not Help	Comment _____

NSAIDS

☐ Ibuprofen (Motrin/Advil)	☐ Helped	☐ Did Not Help	Comment _____
☐ Naproxen (Aleve)	☐ Helped	☐ Did Not Help	Comment _____
☐ Celecoxib (Celebrex)	☐ Helped	☐ Did Not Help	Comment _____
☐ Indomethacin (Indocin)	☐ Helped	☐ Did Not Help	Comment _____
☐ Ketoprofen (Orudis)	☐ Helped	☐ Did Not Help	Comment _____
☐ Meloxicam (Mobic)	☐ Helped	☐ Did Not Help	Comment _____
☐ Other _____	☐ Helped	☐ Did Not Help	Comment _____

Muscle relaxants

☐ Cyclobenzaprine (Flexeril)	☐ Helped	☐ Did Not Help	Comment _____
☐ Tizanidine (Zanaflex)	☐ Helped	☐ Did Not Help	Comment _____
☐ Carisoprodol (Soma)	☐ Helped	☐ Did Not Help	Comment _____
☐ Metaxalone (Skelaxin)	☐ Helped	☐ Did Not Help	Comment _____
☐ Baclofen (Lioresal)	☐ Helped	☐ Did Not Help	Comment _____
☐ Other _____	☐ Helped	☐ Did Not Help	Comment _____

Narcotics

☐ Propoxyphene (Darvocet)	☐ Helped	☐ Did Not Help	Comment _____
☐ Hydrocodone (Vicodin, Lortab)	☐ Helped	☐ Did Not Help	Comment _____
☐ Tramadol (Ultram, Ultracet)	☐ Helped	☐ Did Not Help	Comment _____
☐ Oxycodone (OxyContin, Percocet)	☐ Helped	☐ Did Not Help	Comment _____
☐ Morphine (MS Contin, Kadian)	☐ Helped	☐ Did Not Help	Comment _____
☐ Other _____	☐ Helped	☐ Did Not Help	Comment _____
☐ Other _____	☐ Helped	☐ Did Not Help	Comment _____

Antiseizure medication

☐ Gabapentin (Neurontin)	☐ Helped	☐ Did Not Help	Comment _____
☐ Pregabalin (Lyrica)	☐ Helped	☐ Did Not Help	Comment _____
☐ Topiramate (Topamax)	☐ Helped	☐ Did Not Help	Comment _____

My Neck Hurts!

☐ Levetiracetam (Keppra)	☐ Helped	☐ Did Not Help	Comment _____
☐ Other _____	☐ Helped	☐ Did Not Help	Comment _____

Antidepressants

☐ Duloxetine (Cymbalta)	☐ Helped	☐ Did Not Help	Comment _____
☐ Milnacipran (Savella)	☐ Helped	☐ Did Not Help	Comment _____
☐ Nortriptyline (Pamelor)	☐ Helped	☐ Did Not Help	Comment _____
☐ Amitriptyline (Elavil)	☐ Helped	☐ Did Not Help	Comment _____
☐ Other _____	☐ Helped	☐ Did Not Help	Comment _____

Injection Therapy

☐ Trigger point injection	☐ Helped	☐ Did Not Help	Comment _____
☐ Facet blocks/medial branch blocks	☐ Helped	☐ Did Not Help	Comment _____
☐ RFA (radiofrequency ablation)	☐ Helped	☐ Did Not Help	Comment _____
☐ Occipital nerve blocks	☐ Helped	☐ Did Not Help	Comment _____
☐ Epidurals	☐ Helped	☐ Did Not Help	Comment _____
☐ Botulinum toxin (Botox/Myobloc/ Dysport)	☐ Helped	☐ Did Not Help	Comment _____
☐ Prolotherapy	☐ Helped	☐ Did Not Help	Comment _____
☐ Spinal cord stimulation	☐ Helped	☐ Did Not Help	Comment _____
☐ Other _____	☐ Helped	☐ Did Not Help	Comment _____

Other or alternative treatment not listed

☐ _____	☐ Helped	☐ Did Not Help	Comment _____
☐ _____	☐ Helped	☐ Did Not Help	Comment _____
☐ _____	☐ Helped	☐ Did Not Help	Comment _____

Web Sites

The following Web sites are additional resources for you to consult for more information about the topics discussed in this book. They are listed in an order that corresponds with the sequence of the chapters.

The listing of a Web site in this section should not be considered an endorsement of its content. I encourage you to consult multiple sources of information when researching potential treatment options. When you find a site that is particularly helpful, you can bookmark it and, if desired, share the link with your doctor or therapist.

General Information on Neck Anatomy, Pathology, and Pain Treatment

American College of Rheumatology (information on rheumatological diseases such as arthritis, fibromyalgia, and lupus erythematosus)
www.rheumatology.org

American Pain Society (information on treatments for neck and upper back pain)
www.ampainsoc.org

Neck Pain Care (information on pain conditions and treatments)
www.neckpaincare.com

North American Spine Society (information on spinal health and disease)
www.spine.org

Spine-Health (information on treatments for neck and upper back pain)
www.spine-health.com

Spine Universe (information on treatments for neck and upper back pain)
www.spineuniverse.com

National Pain Foundation (information on pain conditions and treatments)
www.nationalpainfoundation.org

Physical Therapy

About.com: Physical Therapy
www.physicaltherapy.about.com

American Physical Therapy Association
www.apta.org

Electric Stimulation

Empi (information on transcutaneous electrical nerve stimulation units from Empi)
www.empi.com

RS Medical (information on transcutaneous electrical nerve stimulation units and interferential current/muscle stimulation units from RS Medical)
www.rsmedical.com

Vertis PNT (information on percutaneous neuromodulation therapy)
www.pnthealth.com

Manual Therapy

American Academy of Osteopathy
www.academyofosteopathy.org

American Chiropractic Association
www.amerchiro.org

American Massage Therapy Association
www.amtamassage.org

American Osteopathic Association
www.osteopathic.org

Massage Magazine
www.massagemag.com

Medications

RxList (information on medications)
www.rxlist.com

WebMD (information on medications and supplements)
www.webmd.com

Injection Therapy

eOrthopod.com (information on spinal injections)
www.eorthopod.com/public/patient_education/6629/injections_for_pain.html

Neurotoxin Institute (information on multiple uses of botulinum toxin)
www.neurotoxininstitute.com

Complementary and Alternative Therapy

ABC of Yoga
    www.abc-of-yoga.com

American Academy of Medical Acupuncture
    www.medicalacupuncture.org

American Yoga Association
    www.americanyogaassociation.org

Association for Applied Psychophysiology and Biofeedback
    www.aapb.org

National Center for Complementary and Alternative Medicine (government information site on multiple complementary and alternative therapies)
    www.nccam.nih.gov

National Certification Commission for Acupuncture and Oriental Medicine
    www.nccaom.org

Quackwatch (critical reviews of alternative and complementary therapies)
    www.quackwatch.org

Glossary

Acupressure Ancient Chinese treatment involving manually pushing on specific pressure points to balance the body's energy flow and improve health.

Acupuncture An ancient Chinese treatment that uses fine needles to balance the body's energy flow and improve health.

Adjustment Chiropractic term for passive movement of a joint past its normal range of motion to correct a subluxation.

Alexander technique A technique designed to help a person become better aware of his or her balance and posture, meant to improve physical and emotional well-being.

Allopathic physician (M.D.) See *Medical doctor*

Analgesic A substance that relieves pain.

Ankylosing spondylitis A genetic condition that causes the bones of the spine and pelvis to fuse over time.

Annulus fibrosis The outer fibrous layer of an intervertebral disc.

Anterior The front, or ventral, location.

Anticonvulsant A medication designed to prevent seizures that may also be used off-label to treat pain.

Antidepressant A medication designed to treat depression and anxiety that may also be used off-label to treat pain.

Anti-inflammatory A substance that decreases inflammation (e.g., NSAIDs and steroids).

Arnold Chiari malformation A congenital brain abnormality in which a portion of the cerebellum extends through the opening at the base of the skull.

Aromatherapy The use of essential oils to promote health and treat disease.

Biofeedback A technique using electronic monitoring and visual or auditory feedback of the body's responses (breathing, muscle tension, heart rate, sweating) to achieve relaxation and pain relief.

Botulinum toxin Purified protein (Botox, Dysport, or Myobloc) injected into a muscle for the treatment of muscle spasm or pain.

Bulging disc An intervertebral disc that extends beyond its normal anatomical boundaries from a weakening or tear of the outer shell (annulus fibrosis), without extrusion of the inner core (nucleus pulposus).

Capsaicin Topical preparation made from chili peppers used to treat pain.

Central canal Central space formed by the vertebral column filled with the spinal cord, its coverings, and cerebrospinal fluid.

Central nervous system The brain and spinal cord.

Cerebrospinal fluid Fluid surrounding the spinal cord and spinal nerve roots.

Cervical dystonia See *Torticollis.*

Cervical spine The upper portion of the spinal column, made up of seven vertebrae.

Chelation therapy Alternative intravenous treatment with EDTA used to bind excess metals in the blood.

Chiropractor (D.C.) Doctor of chiropractic, trained in the treatment of spinal manipulation.

Coccyx The lowest portion of the vertebral column, also known as the tailbone.

Computer tomography (CT) An x-ray technique with computer enhancement used to create cross-sectional images of the body.

Craniosacral therapy Nontraditional osteopathic technique of subtle skull manipulation.

Discitis Inflammation of an intervertebral disc.

D.O. See *Osteopathic physician.*

Electromyograph (EMG) A diagnostic test used to assess the health of the peripheral nerves and the muscles, typically performed along with nerve conduction studies.

Epidural injections Injections of steroid in the epidural space used to decrease nerve root inflammation. These may be performed with the translaminar or the transforaminal (selective nerve root block) approach.

Facet block (medial branch block) Injection into or around a facet joint to decrease pain and inflammation.

Facet joints Posterior connecting joints between vertebrae.

Fascia The fibrous connective tissue that surrounds muscles.

Feldenkrais method Alternative healing method of healthy movements and breathing to improve self-awareness.

Fibromyalgia Syndrome of clinical symptoms including widespread musculoskeletal pain, specific tender points, fatigue, and sleep disturbance.

Food and Drug Administration (FDA) A government agency that regulates prescription drugs.

Free weights   A type of exercise weight (dumbbell or barbell) used to build muscle strength and bulk.

Herbal therapy   The use of plant extracts to promote health and treat disease.

Herniated disc   Extrusion of the inner core of an intervertebral disc (nucleus pulposus) through a weakness in the outer shell (annulus fibrosis).

Homeopathy   An alternative medical therapy based on the principle of "like cures like." Substances that cause a particular symptom are extremely diluted in water or alcohol to treat that symptom.

Intervertebral disc   Tissues between each vertebral body that work like shock absorbers. Each disc is made of a fibrous outer layer filled with a gel-like center.

Kyphotic   Curvature away from the body seen in the thoracic, sacral, and coccyx spinal regions.

Lamina (laminae)   A portion of a vertebral body that connects the spinous process to the pedicle.

Lordotic   Curvature toward the body seen in the cervical and lumbar spinal regions.

Lumbar spine   Lower portion of the vertebral column, made up of five vertebrae.

Magnetic resonance imaging (MRI)   Diagnostic test that uses powerful magnets to create cross-sectional images of the body.

Magnet therapy   The use of magnets to treat symptoms and disease.

Manipulation   Passive movement of a joint past its normal range of motion.

Manual therapy   Physical manipulation or massage of the musculoskeletal system by a physical therapist, osteopathic physician, chiropractor, or massage therapist.

Massage therapy   See *Therapeutic massage*.

Medial branch block   See *Facet block*.

Medial branch nerve   Sensory nerve to a facet joint.

Medical doctor (M.D.)   Fully licensed physician in the United States able to dispense medicine and perform surgery.

Meridians   The pathways throughout the body for the flow of Qi (energy) reported to be balanced by traditional Chinese acupuncture.

Modalities   Treatments provided as part of a physical therapy program that are primarily topical applications, including hot packs, cold packs, ultrasound, electric stimulation, and traction.

Muscle energy   An osteopathic manual technique in which the patient performs active muscle resistance directed by the physician with the goal of increasing range of motion and decreasing muscle spasm.

Muscle relaxant   Medication that acts on the central nervous system to relax muscles and reduce spasm and pain.

Myelography, myelogram   Diagnostic procedure in which dye is injected into the cerebrospinal fluid in order to image the spinal cord, spinal nerve roots, and intervertebral discs.

Myofascial   Tissue, including muscle and fascia, that helps to support the skeletal system.

Myofascial release   An osteopathic manual technique used to manipulate and stretch the muscles and fascia.

Narcotics   Opioid medications, with addictive potential, used to treat pain.

Nerve conduction studies (NCS)   Diagnostic test performed to assess the health of peripheral nerves, typically performed with electromyography.

Nerve root   Part of a peripheral nerve as it exits the spinal column through a foramen.

Neurologist   A physician (M.D. or D.O.) who specializes in the diagnosis and treatment of diseases and dysfunction of the nervous system.

Neuropathic pain   Pain related to damage or irritation of a nerve.

Neurosurgeon   A surgeon trained to perform brain and spinal surgery.

Nonsteroidal anti-inflammatory drug (NSAID)   A group of medications that have pain-reducing and anti-inflammatory effects.

Nucleus pulposus   Gel-like inner core of a vertebral disc.

Occipital nerve block   An injection at the base of the skull used to treat occipital neuralgia.

Occipital neuralgia   Irritation or inflammation of the occipital nerve, typically causing pain or abnormal sensations at the base of the skull.

Off-label   The use of a medication for a condition not approved by the FDA.

Opioids   See *Narcotics*.

Orthopedic surgeon   A physician (M.D. or D.O.) who specializes in the treatment of diseases and dysfunction of the bones and joints.

Osteoarthritis   Degenerative wear and tear of the joints, also known as degenerative joint disease.

Osteopathic manipulative treatment (OMT)   Techniques of manual manipulation of muscles, soft tissue, and the spine performed by an osteopathic physician.

Osteopathic physician (D.O.)   Fully licensed physician in the United States able to dispense medicine and perform surgery. D.O.s have special training in the musculoskeletal system and manipulation and stress a holistic approach to patient treatment.

Percutaneous neuromodulation therapy (PNT)   An electrical stimulation technique using fine needles to treat neck or back pain.

Peripheral nerves   Nerves outside the central nervous system that transmit and receive information between the spinal cord and brain and parts of the body.

Physiatrist   A physician (M.D. or D.O.) who specializes in physical medicine and rehabilitation.

Physical therapy   Rehabilitation treatment under the direction of a trained health profes-

sional (physical therapist), which can include exercise, stretching, manual therapy, and modalities.

Pilates   An exercise program with the goal of maintaining proper body alignment to stretch and strengthen the muscles.

Pinched nerve   Layman's term typically referring to an irritated or compressed nerve.

Posterior   The back, or dorsal, location.

Qi (pronounced "chee")   The body's energy force manipulated by the treatment of acupuncture.

Radiculopathy   Irritation or damage of a spinal nerve root.

Radiofrequency ablation (RFA)   The use of a heat probe to destroy (ablate) a nerve. For neck pain, this technique can be used to destroy a facet joint's sensory nerve.

Referred pain   Experience of feeling pain distant to the point of origin. For neck pain, this usually means into the arms or head.

Reflexology   Alternative massage-like treatment of the hands and feet to promote health.

Reiki   Alternative Japanese technique that claims to manipulate the body's energy force (Ki).

Rheumatoid arthritis   An autoimmune disease that causes chronic inflammation involving the joints and surrounding tissues.

Rolfing   An alternative method of manual therapy used to separate bound connective tissue.

Sacrum   Triangular bony structure at the base of the lumbar spine that attaches to the pelvis at the sacroiliac joint.

Scoliosis   Abnormal lateral curvature of the spine.

Selective nerve root block   An epidural injection at a specific spinal level.

Selective serotonin reuptake inhibitor (SSRI)   A group of medications approved by the FDA for depression and anxiety that are sometimes used off-label to treat pain.

Spinal cord   Part of the central nervous system located within the spinal canal, primarily in the cervical and thoracic regions, that connects the peripheral nervous system with the brain.

Spinal cord stimulation (SCS)   A treatment therapy that uses electrodes implanted along the spinal cord to block pain impulses from being transmitted to the brain.

Spinal stenosis   A reduction in diameter, or narrowing, of the spinal column's central canal.

Spinous process   Posterior portion of a vertebra that connects to the lamina.

Spondylolisthesis   Slippage or displacement of one vertebra on another related to trauma or spondylolysis.

Spondylolysis   A defect in the posterior portion of the vertebra that connects the spinous process with the facet joint.

Spondylosis   Degeneration of the spinal vertebra, causing "spurs," or thickening of the bone.

Sprain   An injury resulting from overstretching or tearing of a ligament.

Strain   An injury resulting from overstretching or tearing of a muscle or tendon.

Subluxation   A term used by chiropractors to describe a misalignment of a vertebra that may be palpated but cannot be seen on an x-ray.

Symptom   A physical or emotional complaint.

Systemic lupus erythematosus   An autoimmune disease that causes chronic inflammation and may affect multiple tissues, including the skin, joints, and kidneys.

Tai Chi   Ancient mind-body practice similar to yoga.

Tender point   Local area of muscle that is tender to the touch, occurring in multiple locations and not causing referred pain. Seen in fibromyalgia.

Therapeutic massage (massage therapy)   Manual manipulation of the muscles and soft tissue to promote relaxation and to reduce muscle tightness and pain.

Therapeutic touch   Alternative therapy that claims to balance a person's energy field to promote health.

Thoracic spine   Midportion of the spinal column, made up of twelve vertebrae.

Titration   Increasing the dose of a medication slowly to avoid side effects and to achieve a higher or therapeutic level.

Topical   Applied to the skin.

Torticollis (cervical dystonia)   Abnormal spontaneous twisting and contracting of the cervical musculature, also known as a wry neck.

Traction   A linear pulling force or stretching of the spine that may be performed manually or with a device.

Transverse process   Portion of a vertebra that projects laterally.

Tricyclic antidepressant   A group of medications approved by the FDA for the treatment of depression and commonly used off-label for pain and sleep problems.

Trigger point   Hyperirritable point in a muscle that, when touched, feels like a taut band and causes referred pain. Seen in myofascial pain.

Vertebrae   Plural of vertebra. The bones that make up the spinal column.

Vertebral body   Main bony portion of a vertebra that supports the vertebral column along with the intervertebral discs.

Wong-Baker FACES Pain Rating Scale   A series of drawings of simplified facial expressions, developed to rate pain for adults and children over age three.

X-ray (radiography)   The use of x-ray beams to visualize an object. In medicine this technique is most commonly used to visualize the bones of the body.

Yoga   A system of physical exercise and stretching with breathing and meditation techniques that is performed to enhance spiritual and physical well-being.

Index

neural foramen, 5, 8

neurologists, 28, 146–47

Neurontin, 96, 97

neuropathic pain, 74

neurosurgeons, 148

norepinephrine and serotonin antagonists, 99

norepinephrine-dopamine reuptake inhibitors, 98

Norflex or Norgesic, 100

Norpramin, 98

nortriptyline, 98

notebooks, taking to appointments, 4

NSAIDs (nonsteroidal anti-inflammatory drugs), 19, 92–94

nucleus pulposus, 8

Nucynta, 100

Nuprin, 93

occipital nerve blocks, 111–13

occipital neuralgia, 26–27, 111

off-label medication use, 97

Opana, 95

opioids, 94–96, 100–101

orphenadrine citrate, 100

orthopedic surgeons, 147–48

Orudis, 93

Oruvail, 93

osteoarthritis, 19–20

osteopathic manipulative treatment (OMT), 83–86

osteopathic physicians, 83–84, 89, 126

over-ball W exercises, 50

overhead presses, 52

oxaprozin, 93

oxcarbazepine, 96

oxycodone, 95

OxyContin, 95

oxymorphone, 95

pain: breakthrough, 94; cycle of, 142–43; long-term or chronic, definition of, x; myofascial, 22–23, 25; neuropathic, 74; psychosocial factors of, 27–29; ratings

and descriptions of, 14–17; referred, 23. *See also* causes of pain

pain questionnaire, 150–53

Pamelor, 98

Parafon Forte or Paraflex, 100

paroxetine, 98

patient questionnaire, 150–53

patient stories: Botox injections, 109–10; cervical traction, 64–65; description of, xi; facet injections, 148–49; injection therapy, 112–13, 115–16; massage, 82; physical therapy, 35, 53; PNT, 73–74

Paxil, 98

pectoralis major stretches, 39

pectoralis minor stretches, 39

Percocet, 94, 95

Percodan, 95

percutaneous neuromodulation therapy (PNT), 69–74

peripheral nerve, 31

phonophoresis, 61

physiatrists, 146

physical therapy: aquatherapy, 53–58; band and body ball therapy, 47–52; cervical traction, 62–65; cold and ice packs, 61; electrical stimulation, 62; ergonomics, 58–59; exercise, 36–46; free weights, 50–52; heat packs, 60; iontophoresis and phonophoresis, 61; manual therapy, 65; overview of, 33–34, 65; posture, 58–59; resources on, 156; strengthening exercises, 41–45; stretching exercises, 36–40; ultrasound, 59; whiplash and, 19

physicians. *See* doctors

Pilates, 129–31

piroxicam, 93

PNT (percutaneous neuromodulation therapy), 69–74

Ponstel, 93

posterior longitudinal ligaments, 9

posterior scalene stretches, 38

posture, 58–59

pregabalin, 96, 97

pressure point therapy (Shiatsu), 80–81